THANK YOU FOR YOUR CONTINUED SUPPORT.

Published By My Littl' Workshop

To purchase additional
copies of this book, go to:
www.MyLittlWorkshop.com

My Littl' Workshop supports Sista Foundation Inc. a nonprofit which empowers young women and mentoring young men, and communities at large through workshops and social events.

This Recipe Book Belongs To

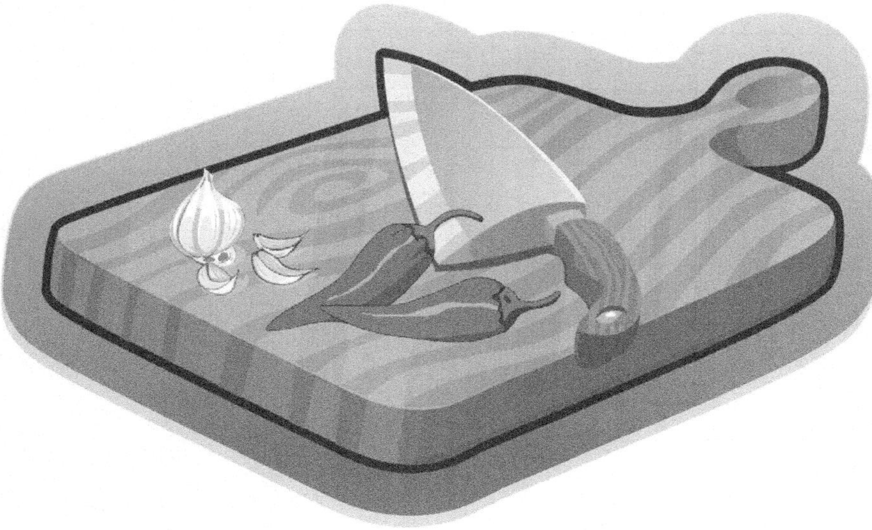

RECIPE:

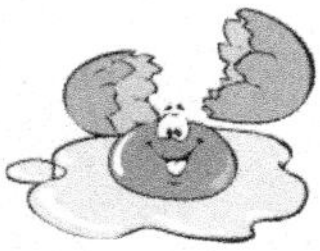

Cooking Instructions

Ingredients

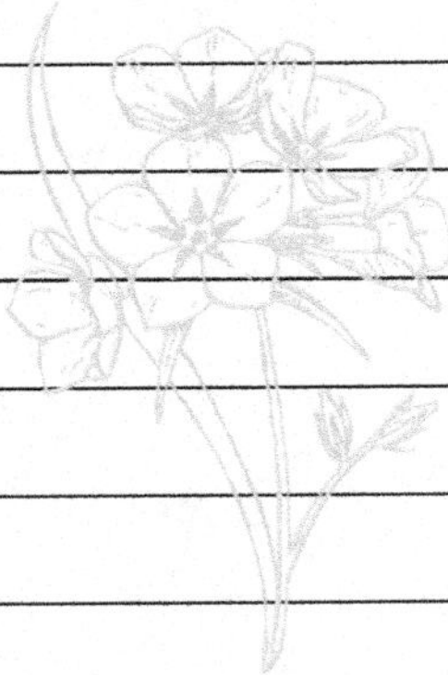

Allergens

RECIPE:

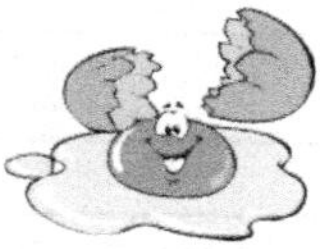

Cooking Instructions

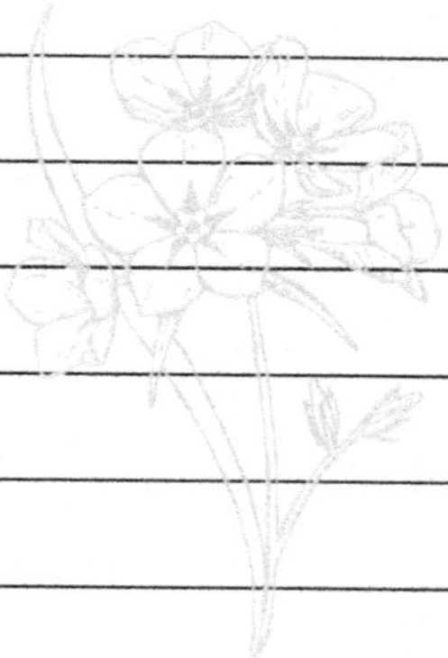

Ingredients

Allergens

RECIPE:

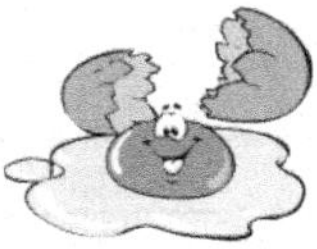

Cooking Instructions

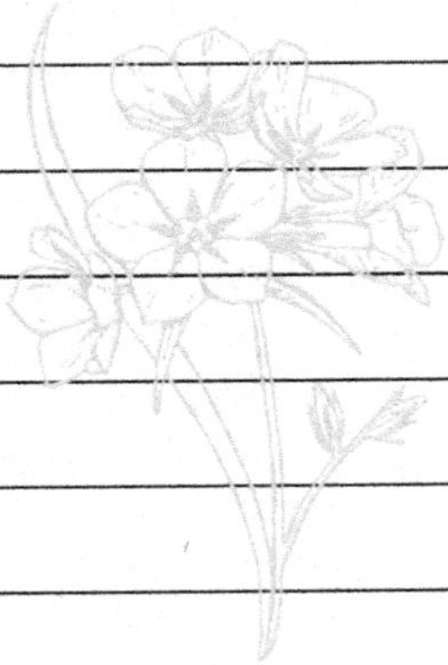

Ingredients

Allergens

RECIPE:

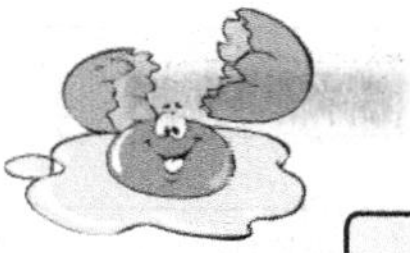

Cooking Instructions

Ingredients

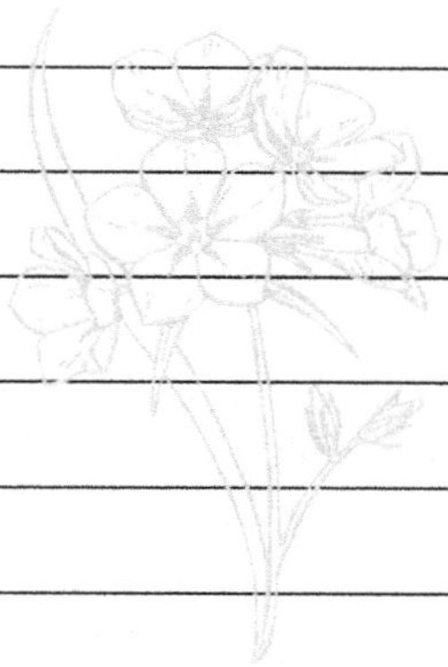

Allergens

RECIPE:

Cooking Instructions

Ingredients

Allergens

RECIPE:

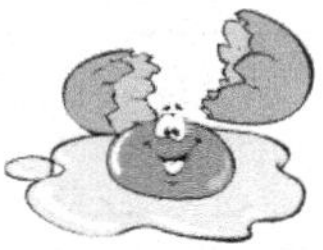

Cooking Instructions

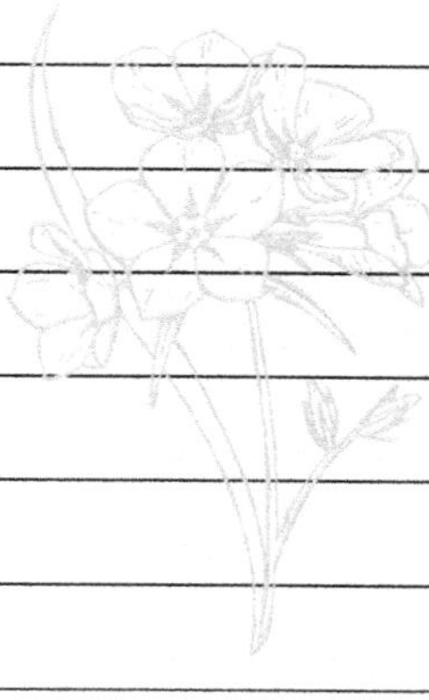

Ingredients

Allergens

RECIPE:

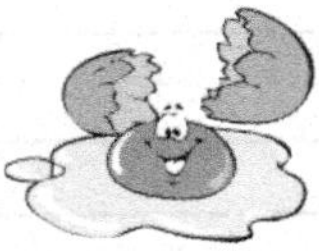

Cooking Instructions

Ingredients

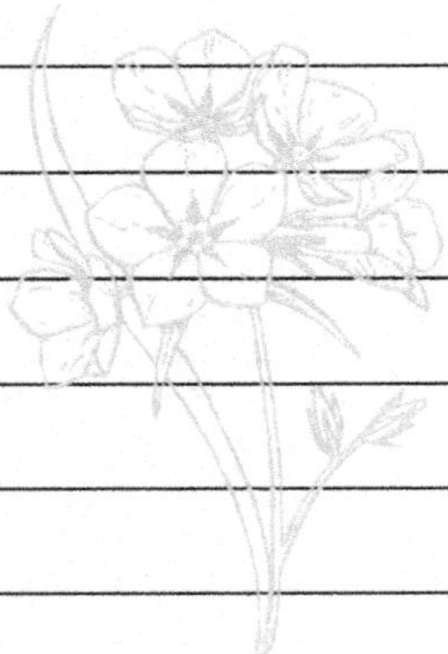

Allergens

RECIPE:

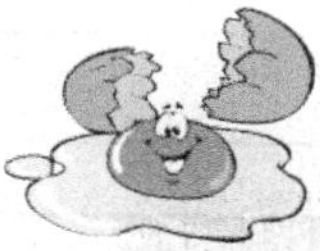

Cooking Instructions

Ingredients

Allergens

RECIPE:

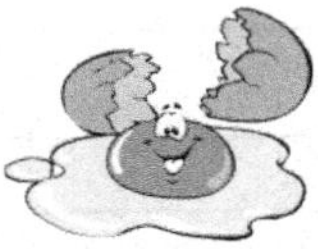

Cooking Instructions

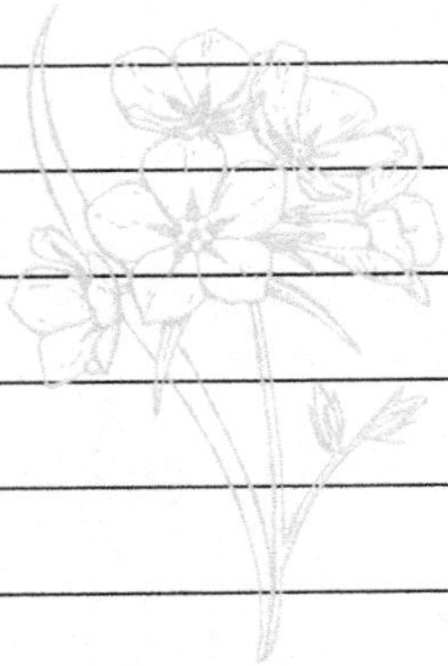

Ingredients

Allergens

RECIPE:

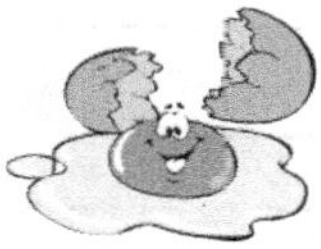

Cooking Instructions

Ingredients

Allergens

RECIPE:

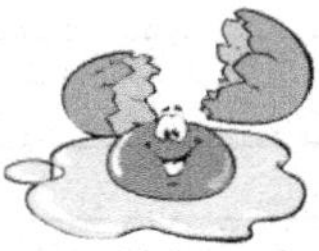

Cooking Instructions

Ingredients

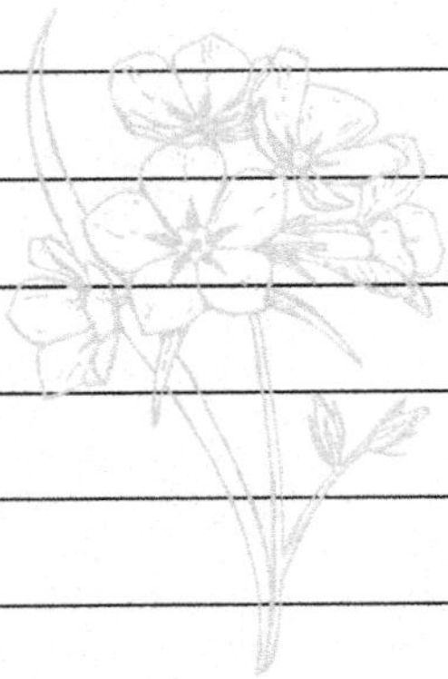

Allergens

RECIPE:

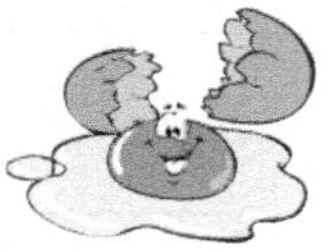

Cooking Instructions

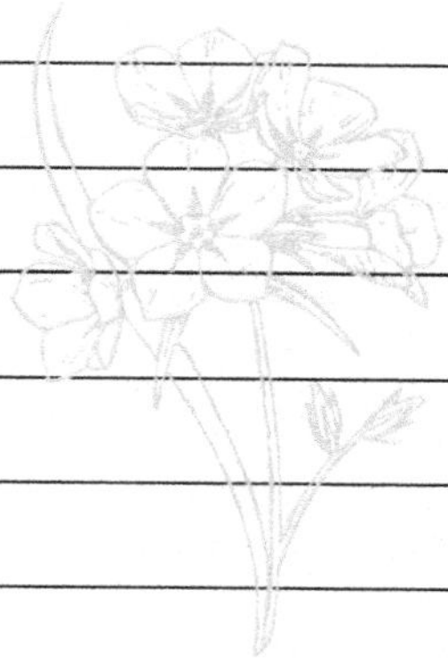

Ingredients

Allergens

RECIPE:

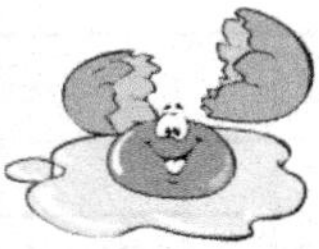

Cooking Instructions

Ingredients

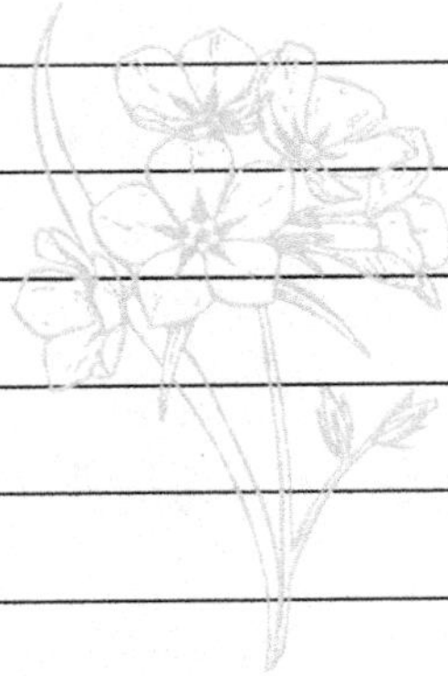

Allergens

RECIPE:

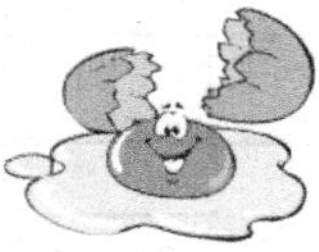

Cooking Instructions

Ingredients

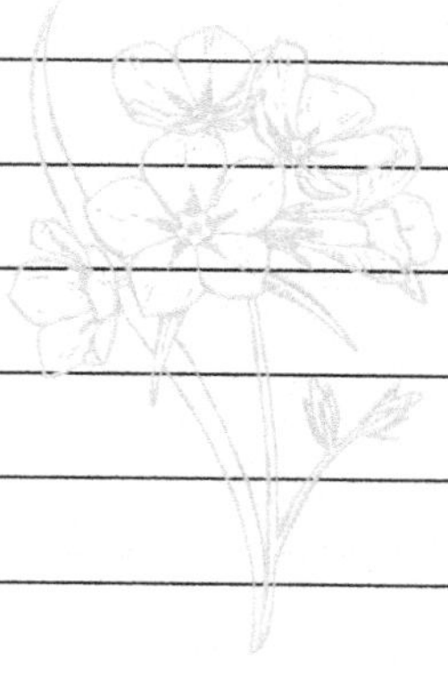

Allergens

RECIPE:

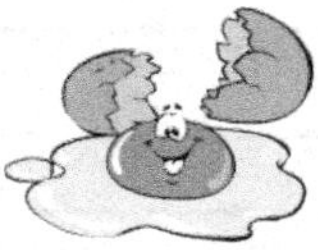

Cooking Instructions

Ingredients

Allergens

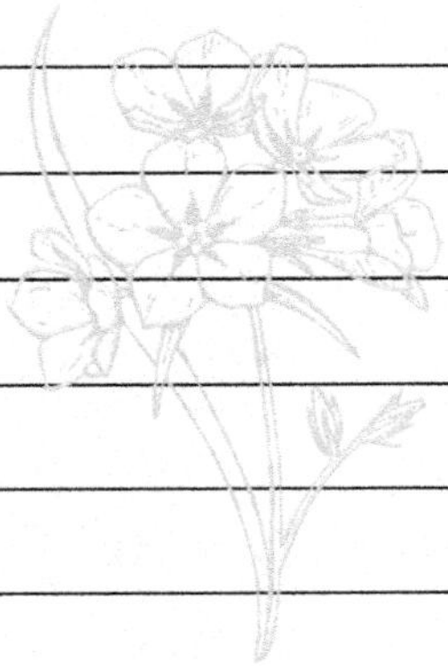

RECIPE:

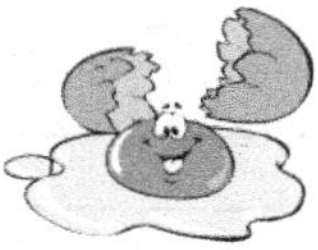

Cooking Instructions

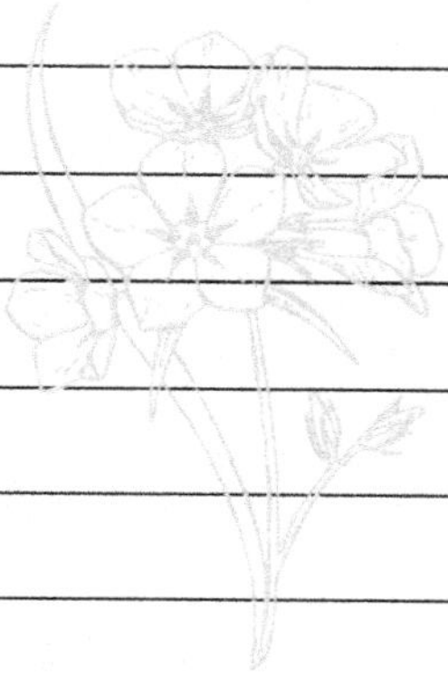

Ingredients

Allergens

RECIPE:

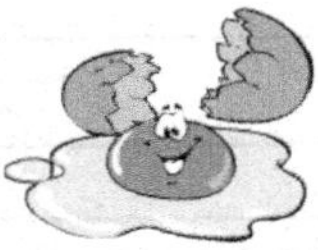

Cooking Instructions

Ingredients

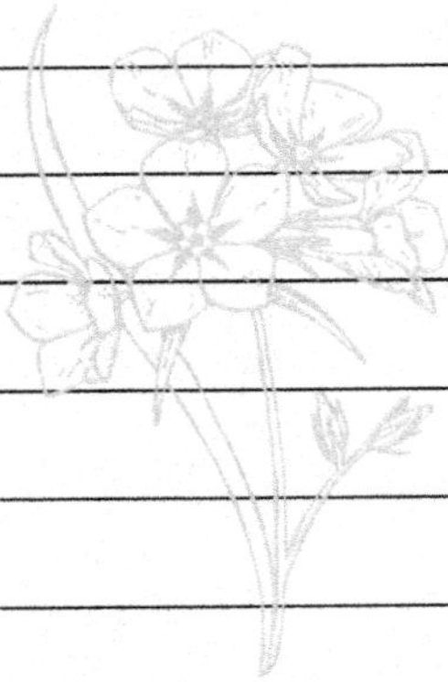

Allergens

RECIPE:

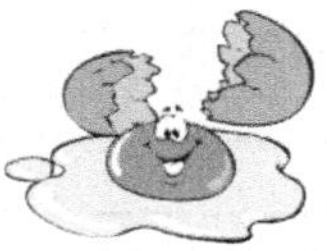

Cooking Instructions

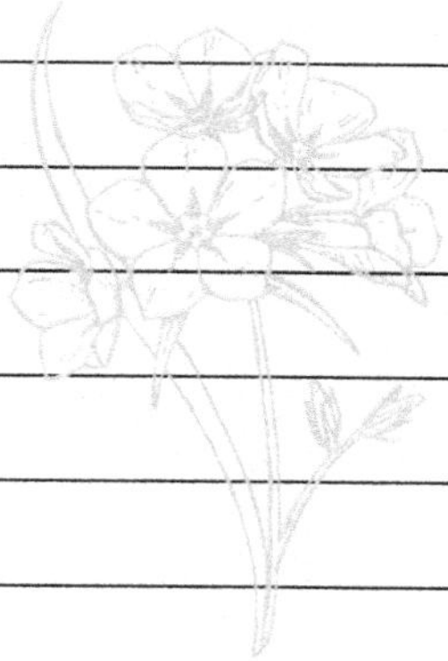

Ingredients

Allergens

RECIPE:

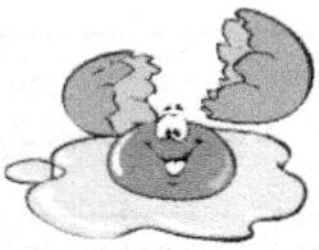

Cooking Instructions

Ingredients

Allergens

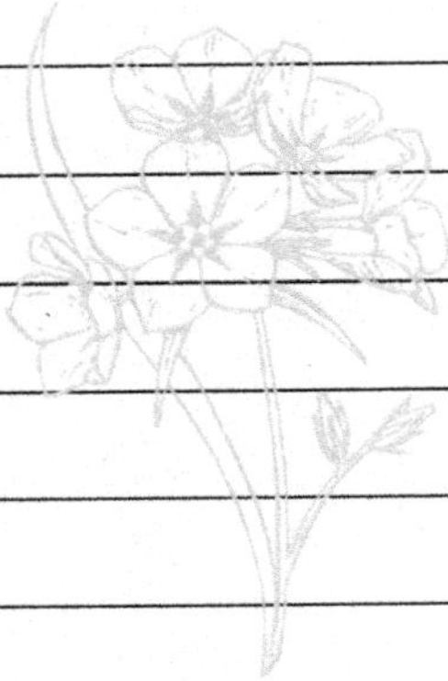

RECIPE:

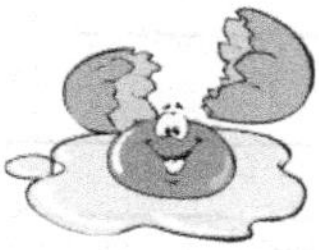

Cooking Instructions

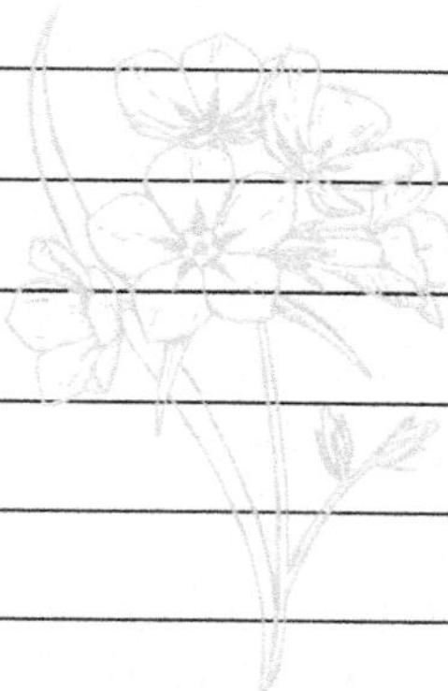

Ingredients

Allergens

RECIPE:

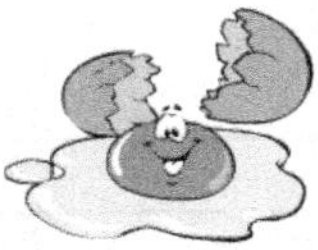

Cooking Instructions

Ingredients

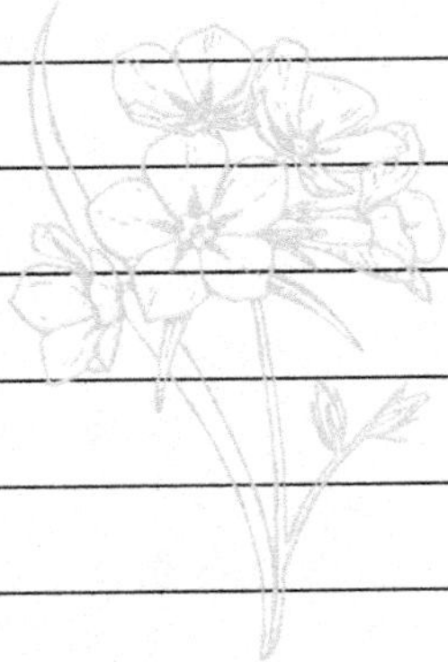

Allergens

RECIPE:

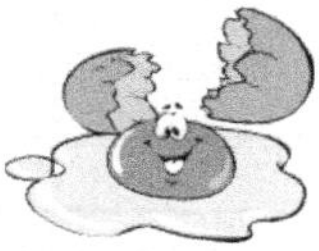

Cooking Instructions

Ingredients

Allergens

RECIPE:

Cooking Instructions

Ingredients

Allergens

RECIPE:

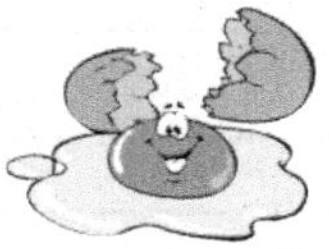

Cooking Instructions

Ingredients

Allergens

RECIPE:

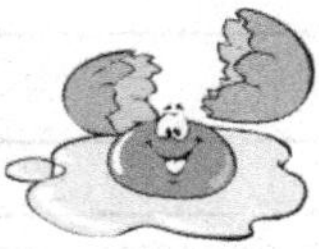

Cooking Instructions

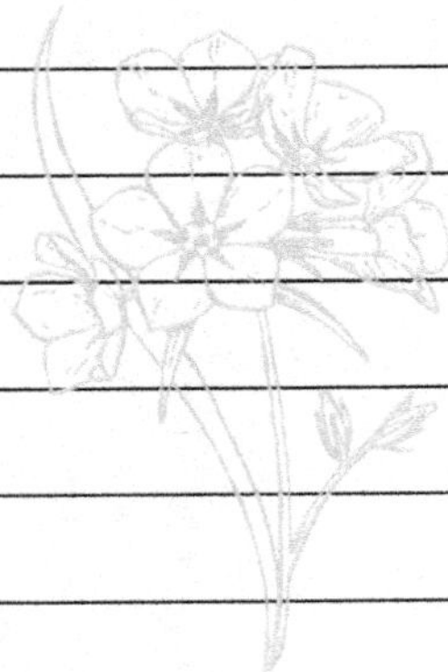

Ingredients

Allergens

RECIPE:

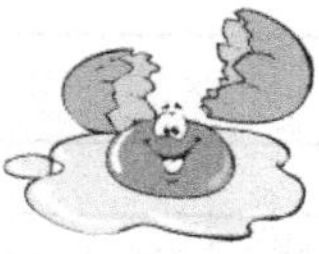

Cooking Instructions

Ingredients

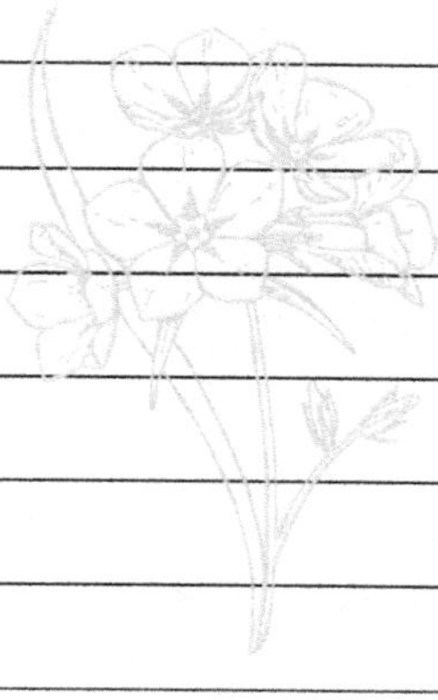

Allergens

RECIPE:

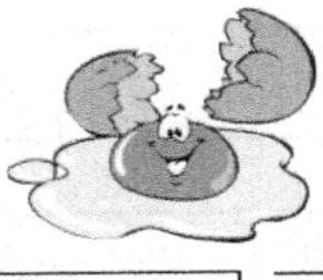

Cooking Instructions

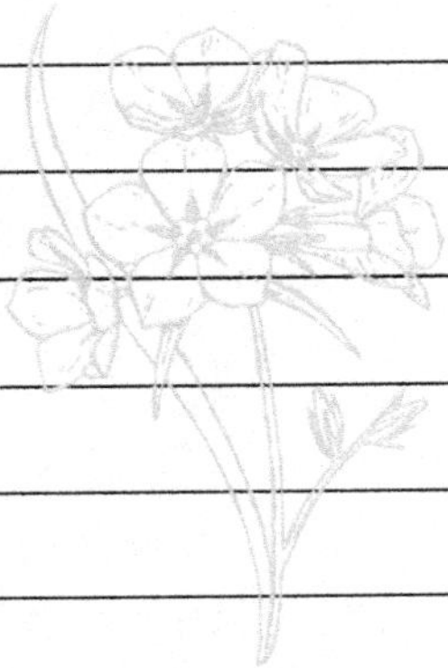

Ingredients

Allergens

RECIPE:

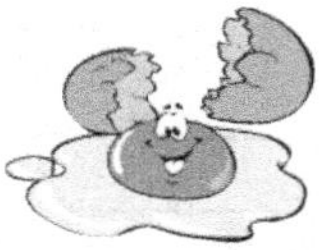

Cooking Instructions

Ingredients

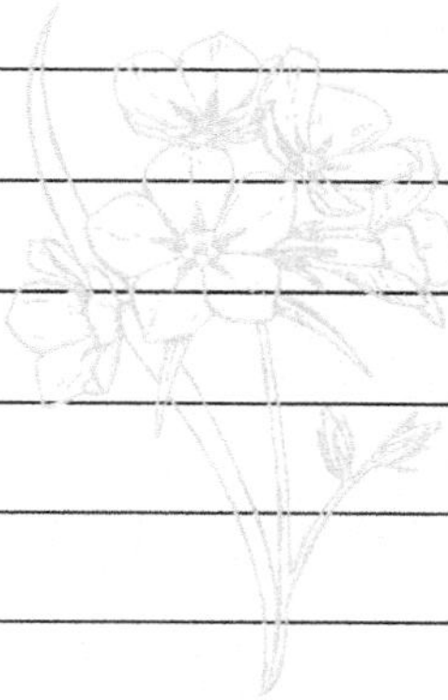

Allergens

RECIPE:

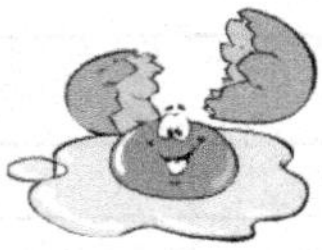

Cooking Instructions

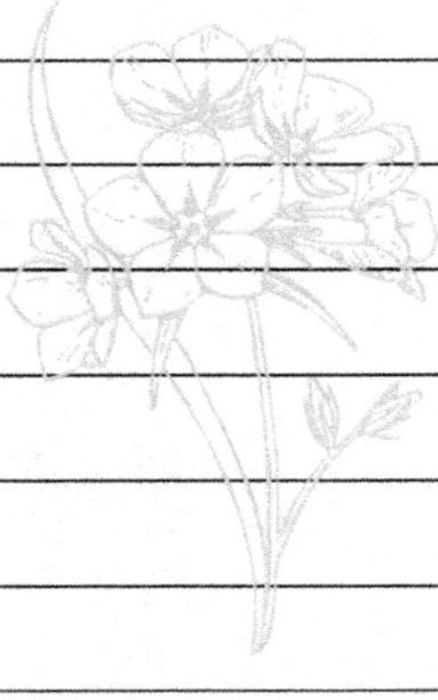

Ingredients

Allergens

RECIPE:

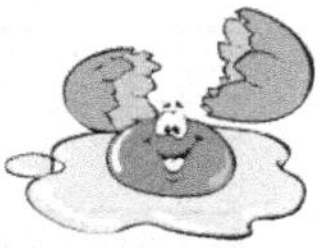

Cooking Instructions

Ingredients

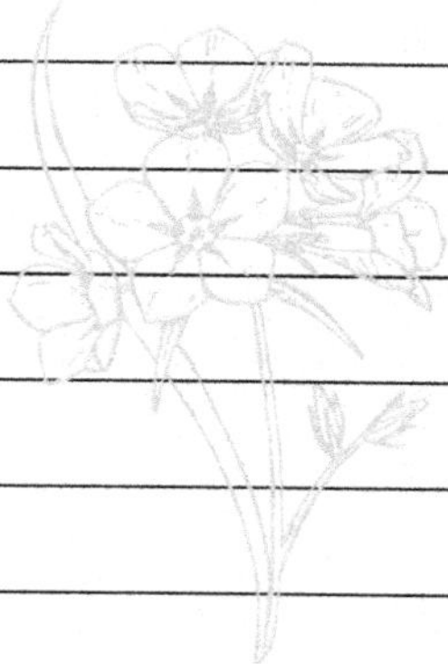

Allergens

RECIPE:

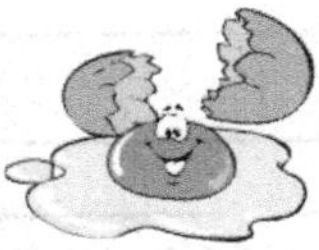

Cooking Instructions

Ingredients

Allergens

RECIPE:

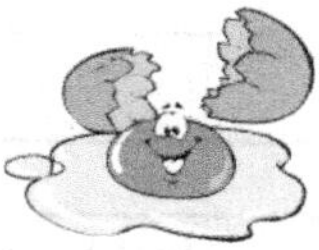

Cooking Instructions

Ingredients

Allergens

RECIPE:

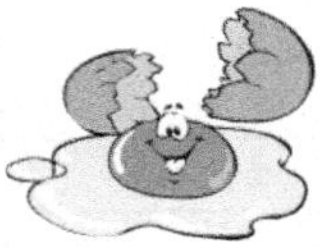

Cooking Instructions

Ingredients

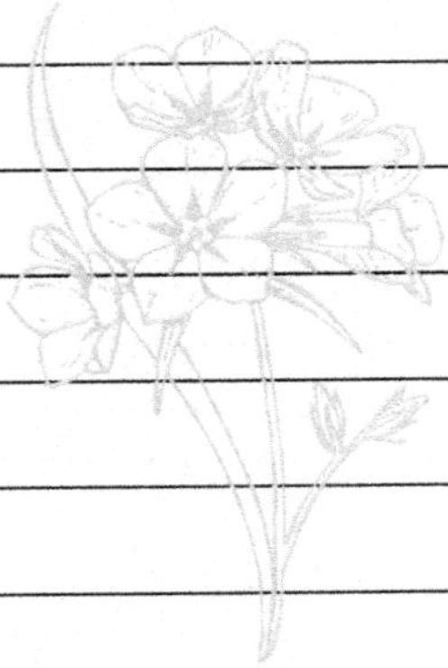

Allergens

RECIPE:

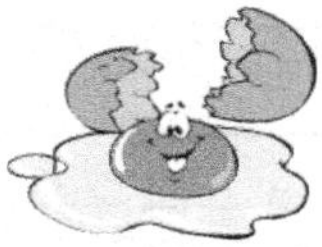

Cooking Instructions

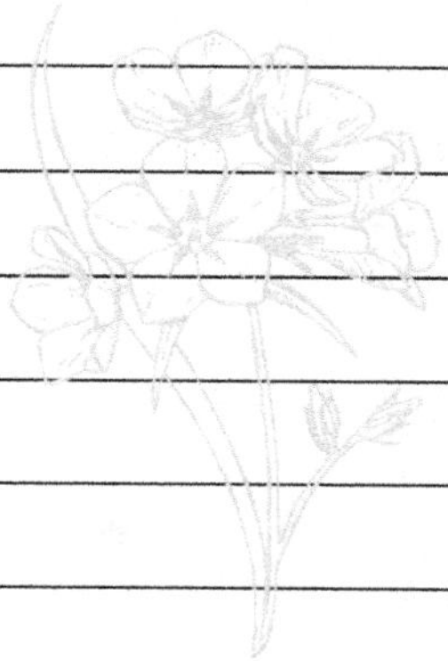

Ingredients

Allergens

RECIPE:

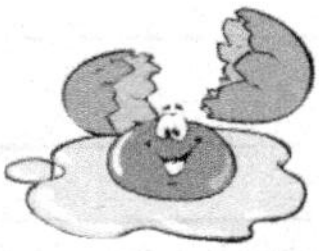

Cooking Instructions

Ingredients

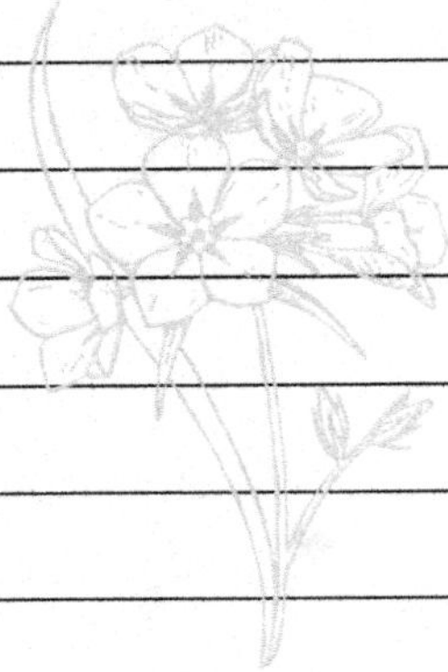

Allergens

RECIPE:

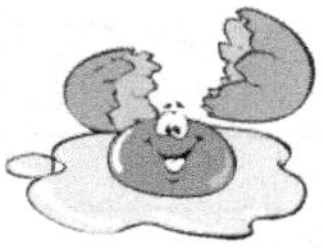

Cooking Instructions

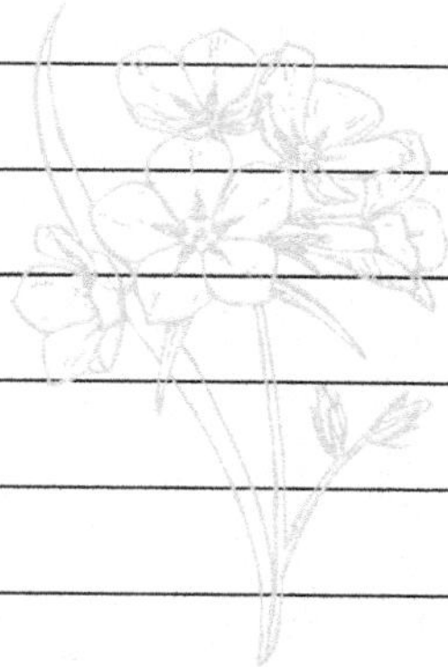

Ingredients

Allergens

RECIPE:

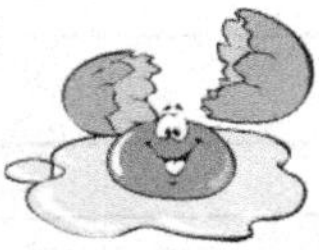

Cooking Instructions

Ingredients

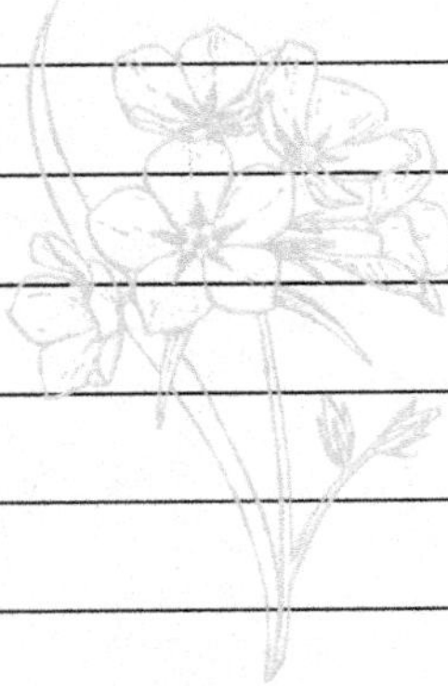

Allergens

RECIPE:

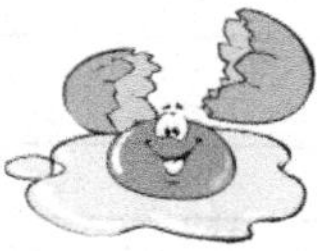

Cooking Instructions

Ingredients

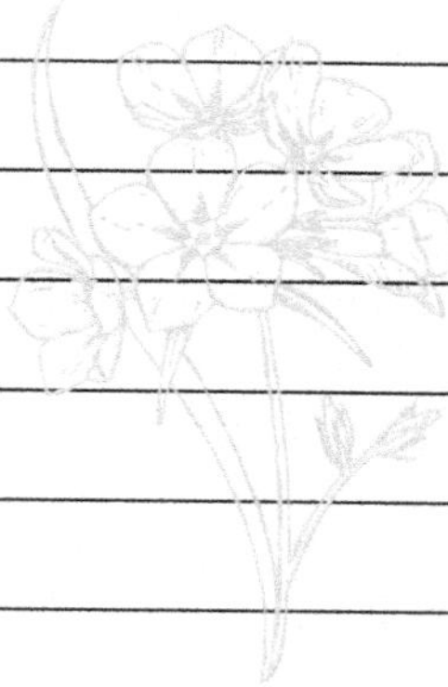

Allergens

RECIPE:

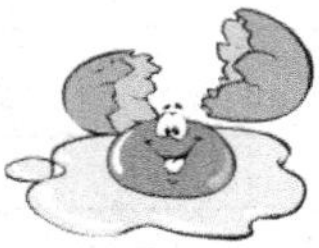

Cooking Instructions

Ingredients

Allergens

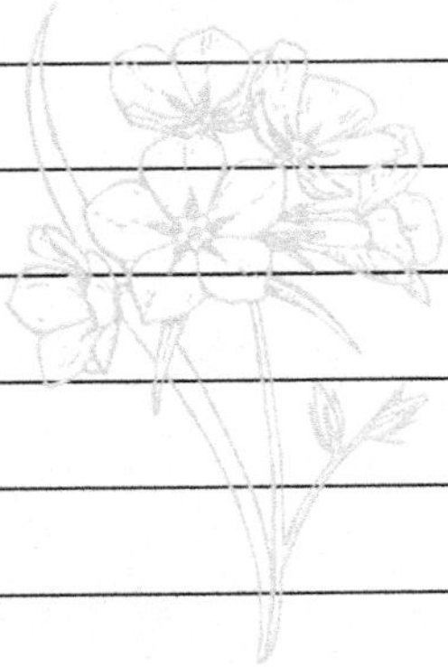

RECIPE:

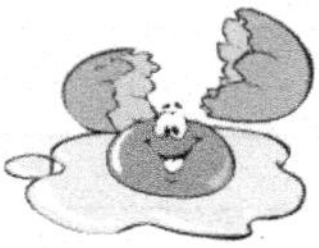

Cooking Instructions

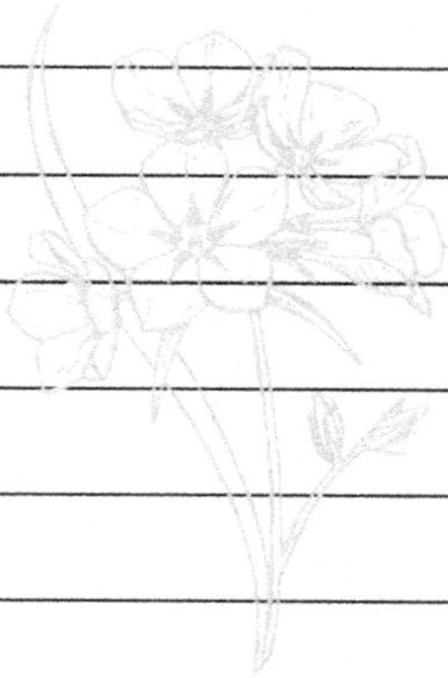

Ingredients

Allergens

RECIPE:

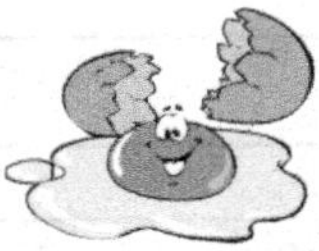

Cooking Instructions

Ingredients

Allergens

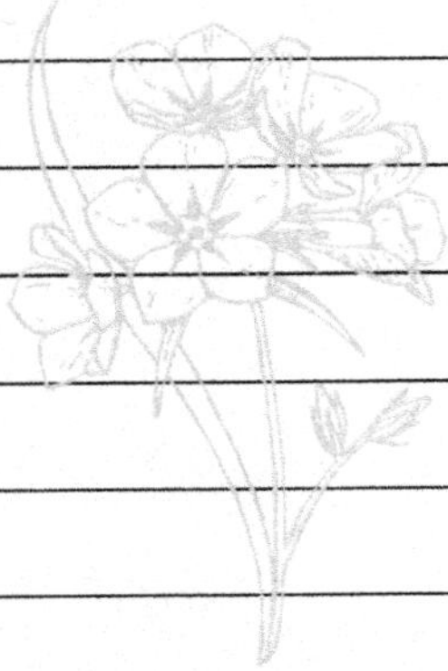

RECIPE:

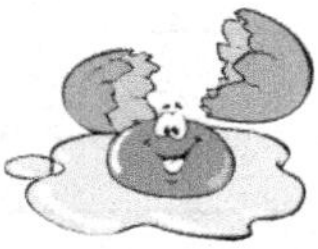

Cooking Instructions

Ingredients

Allergens

RECIPE:

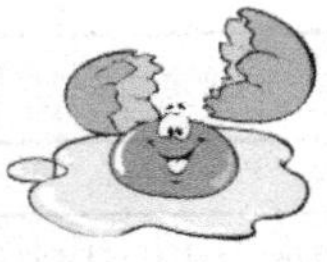

Cooking Instructions

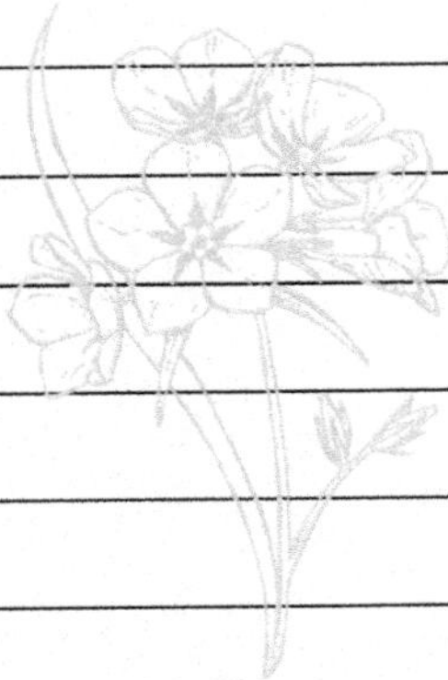

Ingredients

Allergens

RECIPE:

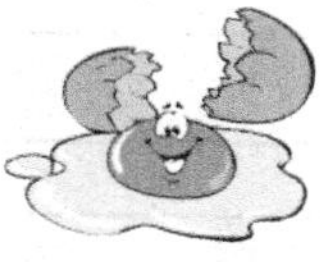

Cooking Instructions

Ingredients

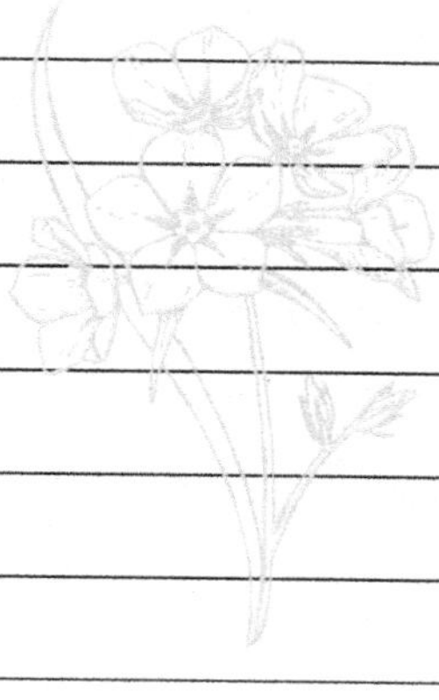

Allergens

RECIPE:

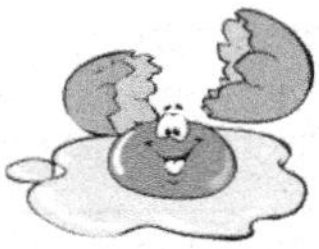

Cooking Instructions

Ingredients

Allergens

RECIPE:

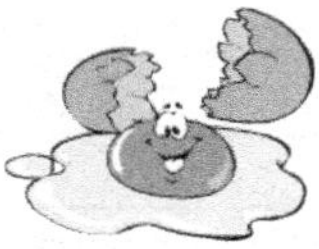

Cooking Instructions

Ingredients

Allergens

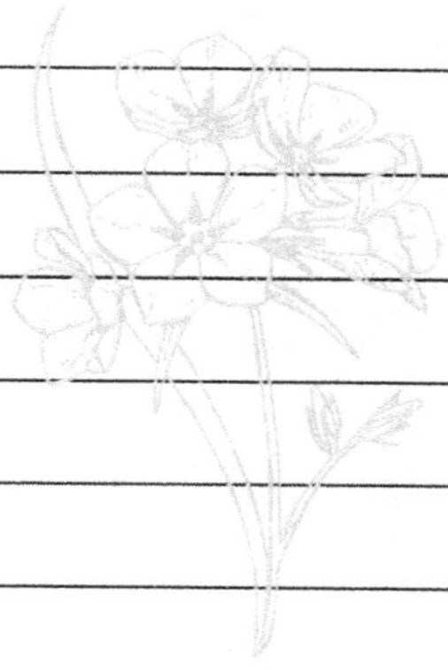

RECIPE:

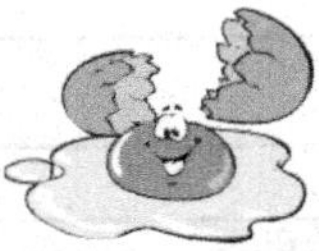

Cooking Instructions

Ingredients

Allergens

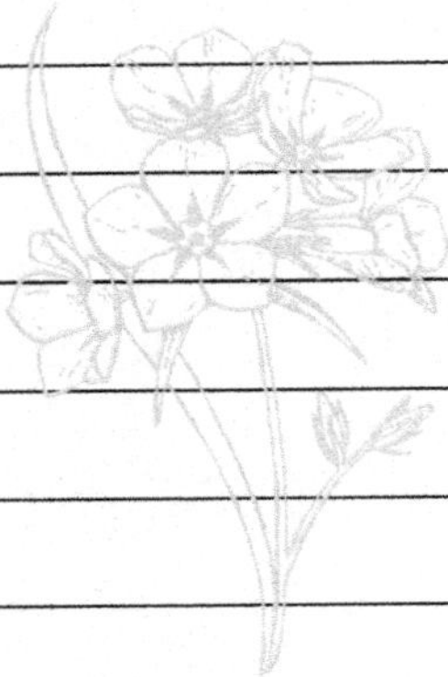

RECIPE:

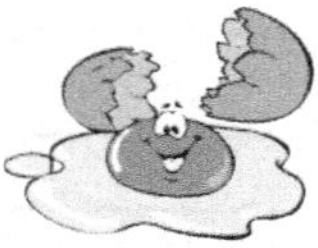

Cooking Instructions

Ingredients

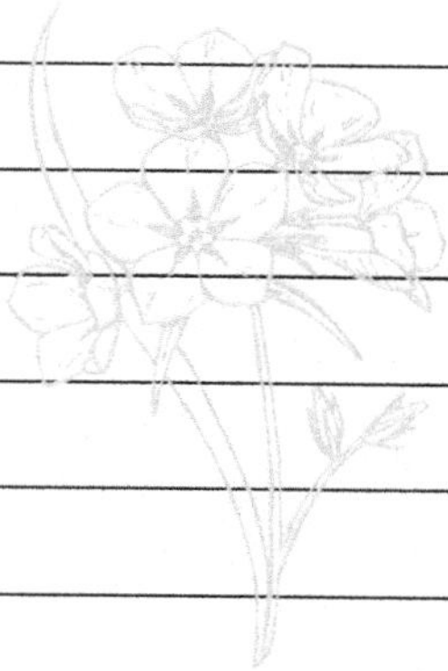

Allergens

RECIPE:

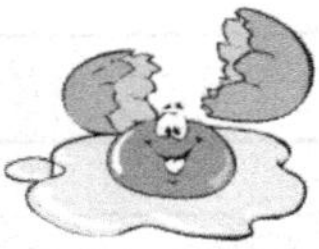

Cooking Instructions

Ingredients

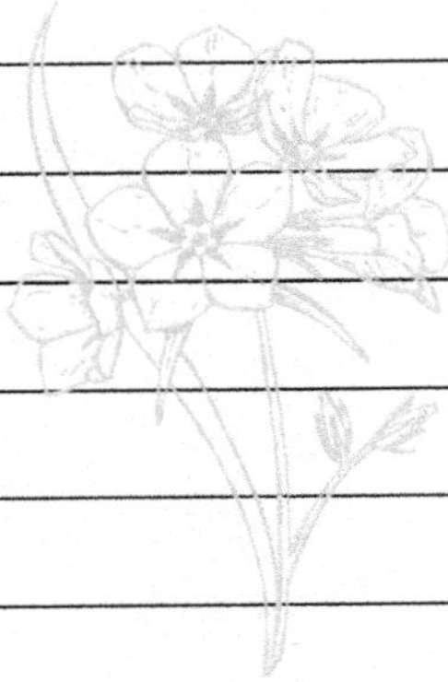

Allergens

RECIPE:

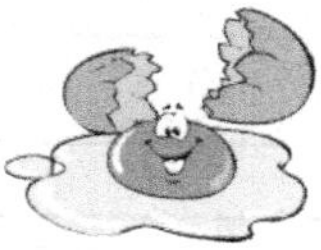

Cooking Instructions

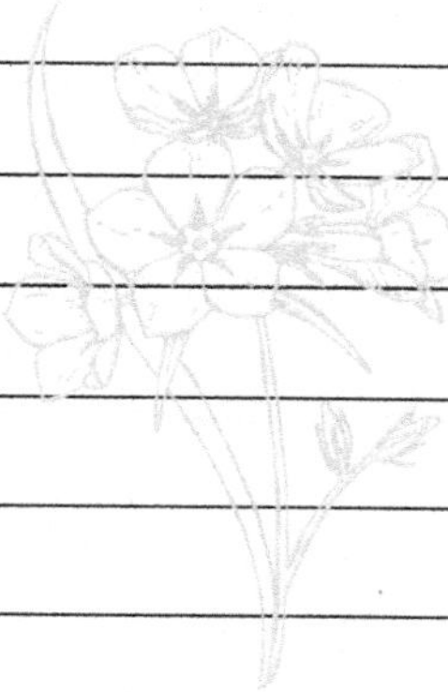

Ingredients

Allergens

RECIPE:

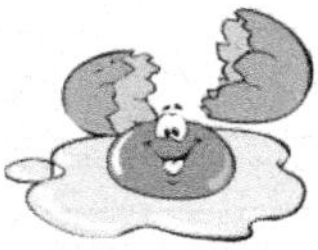

Cooking Instructions

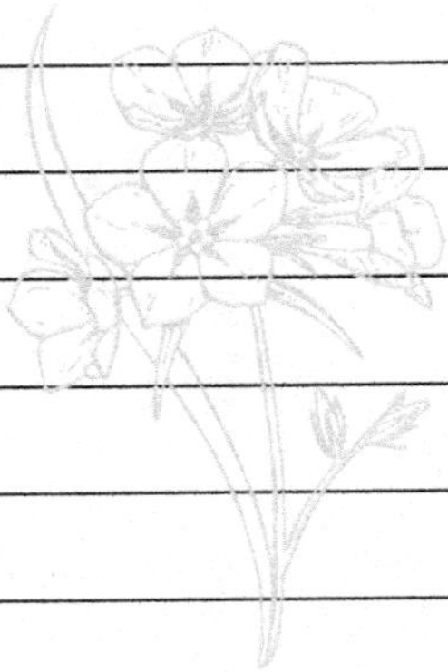

Ingredients

Allergens

RECIPE:

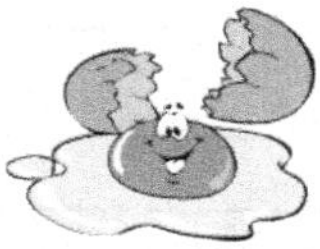

Cooking Instructions

Ingredients

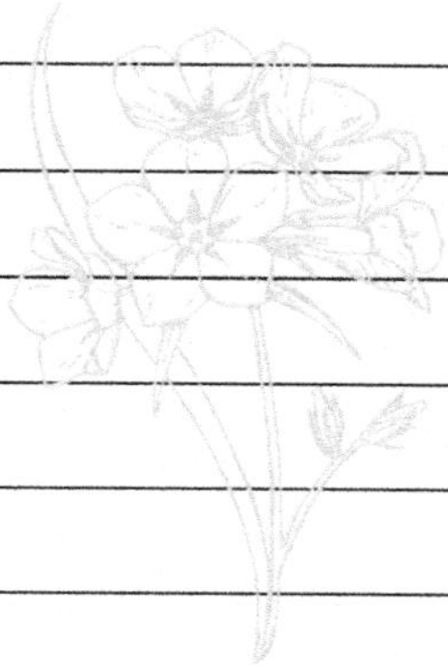

Allergens

RECIPE:

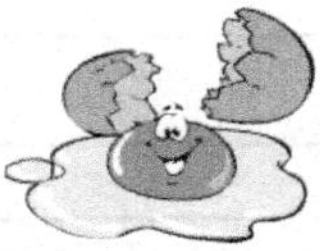

Cooking Instructions

Ingredients

Allergens

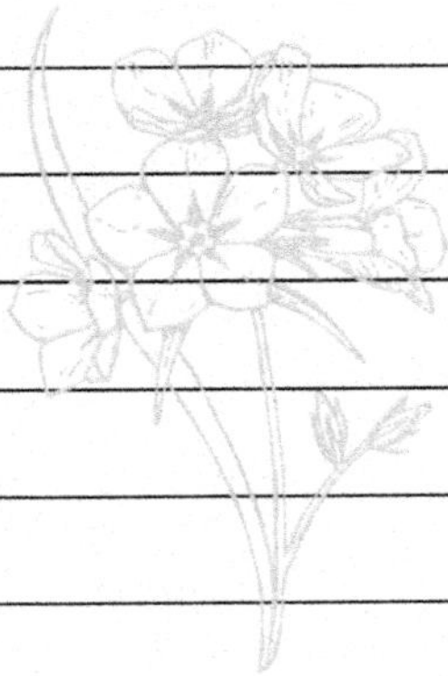

RECIPE:

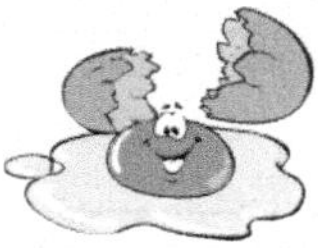

Cooking Instructions

Ingredients

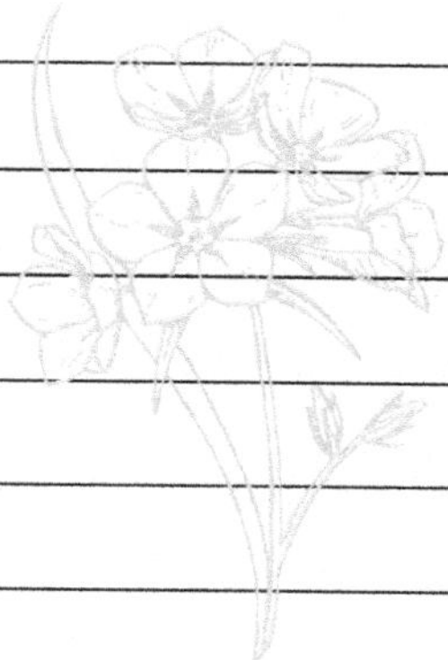

Allergens

RECIPE:

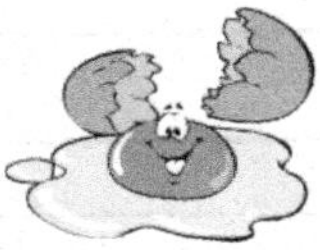

Cooking Instructions

Ingredients

Allergens

RECIPE:

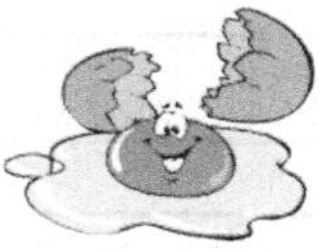

Cooking Instructions

Ingredients

Allergens

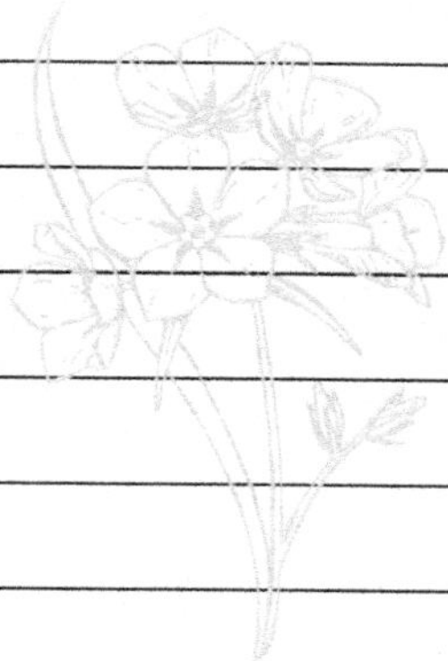

RECIPE:

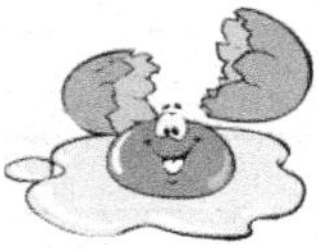

Cooking Instructions

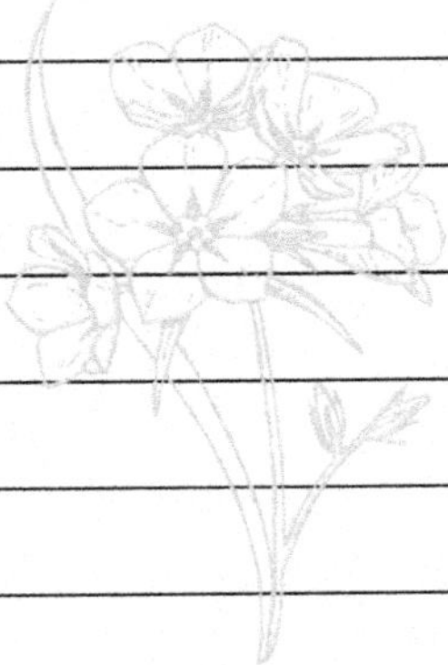

Ingredients

Allergens

RECIPE:

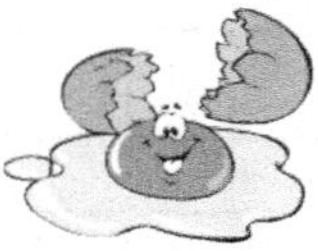

Cooking Instructions

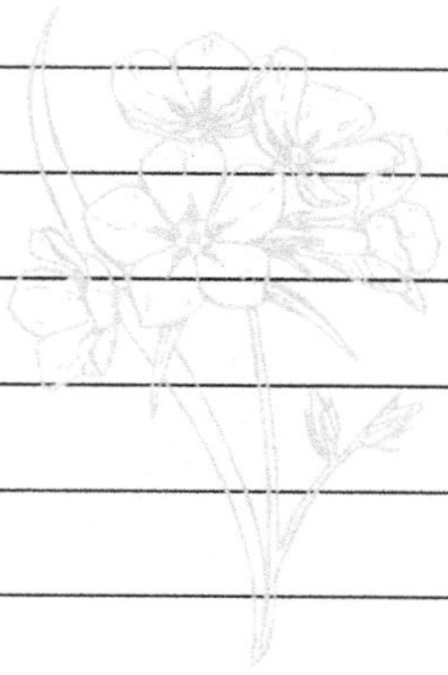

Ingredients

Allergens

RECIPE:

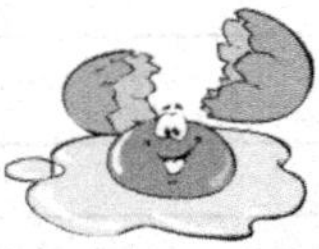

Cooking Instructions

Ingredients

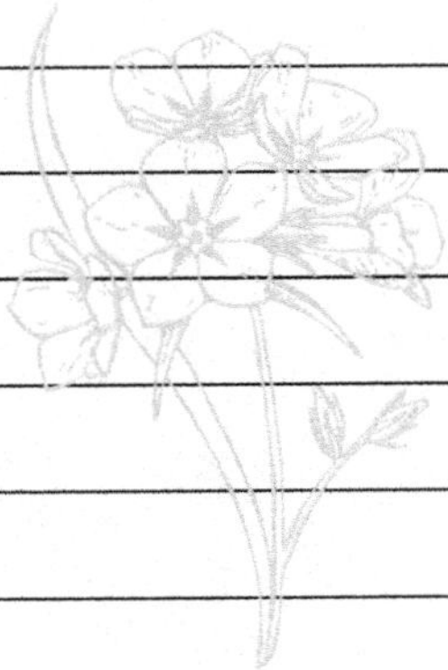

Allergens

RECIPE:

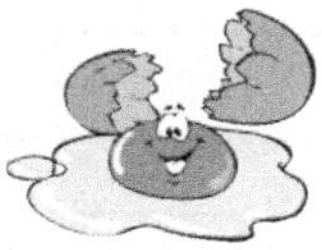

Cooking Instructions

Ingredients

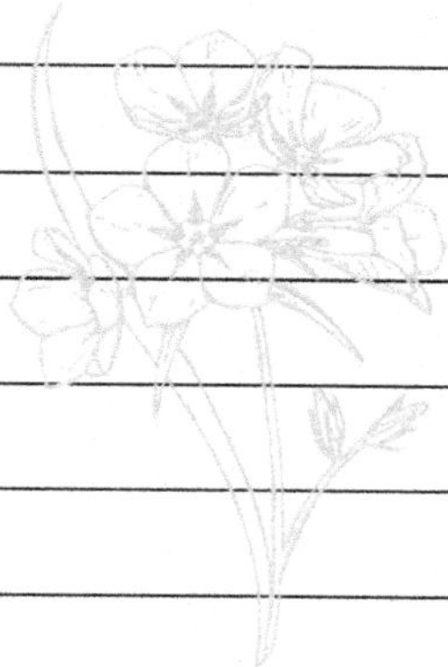

Allergens

RECIPE:

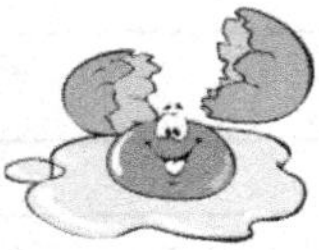

Cooking Instructions

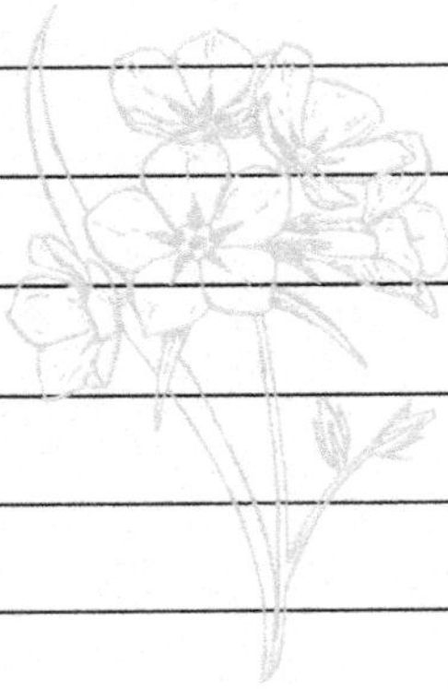

Ingredients

Allergens

RECIPE:

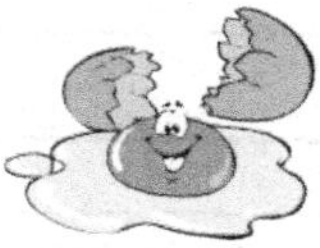

Cooking Instructions

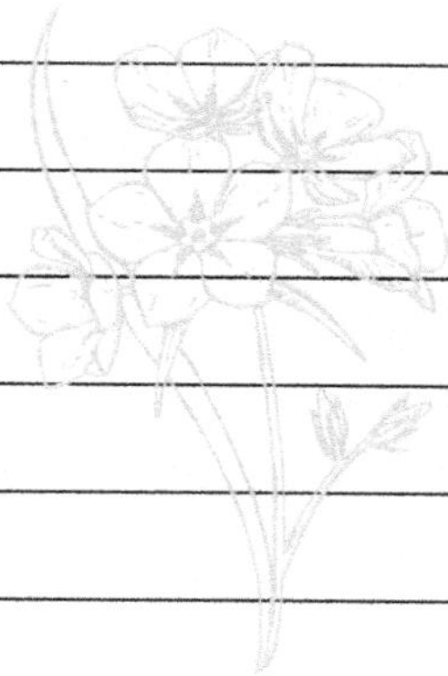

Ingredients

Allergens

RECIPE:

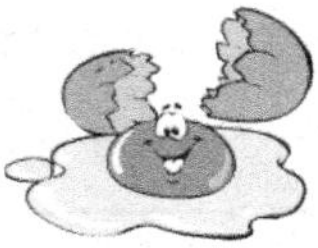

Cooking Instructions

Ingredients

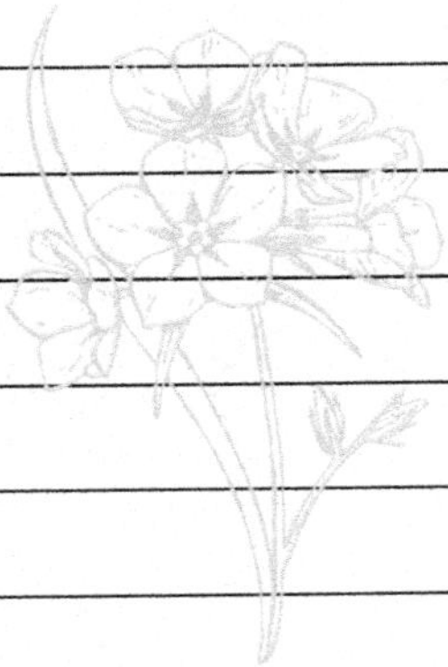

Allergens

RECIPE:

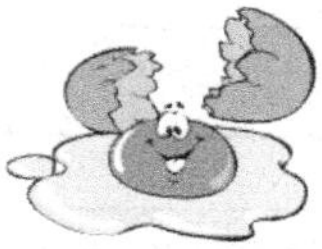

Cooking Instructions

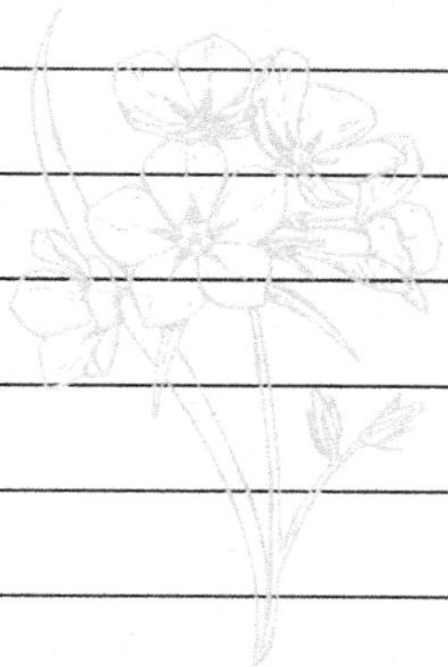

Ingredients

Allergens

RECIPE:

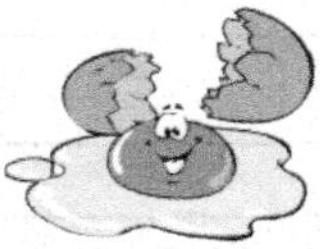

Cooking Instructions

Ingredients

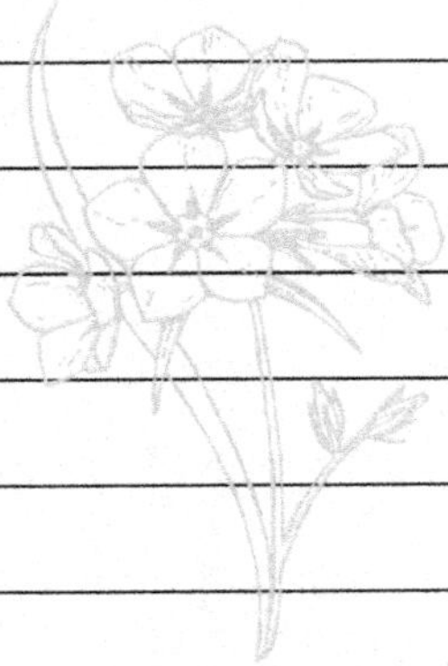

Allergens

RECIPE:

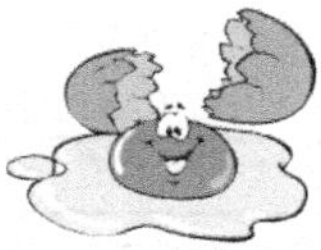

Cooking Instructions

Ingredients

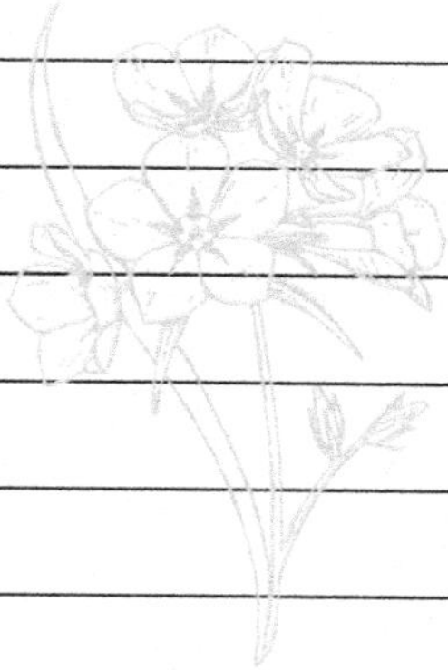

Allergens

RECIPE:

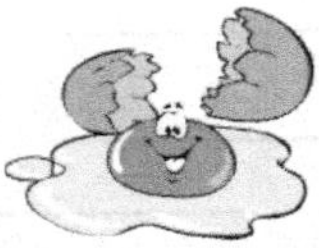

Cooking Instructions

Ingredients

Allergens

RECIPE:

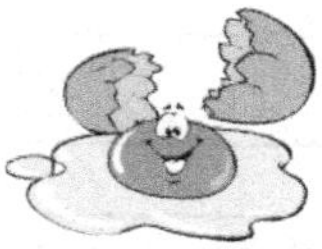

Cooking Instructions

Ingredients

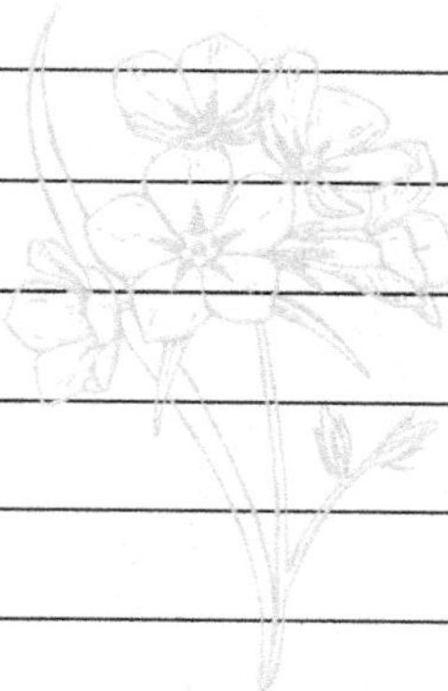

Allergens

RECIPE:

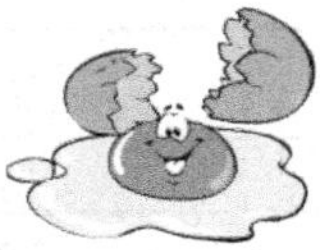

Cooking Instructions

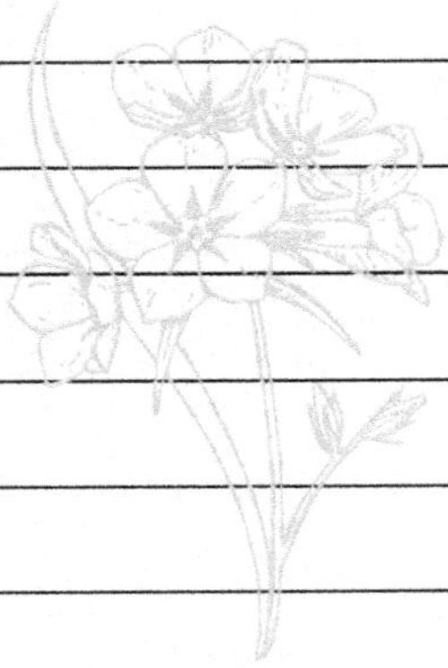

Ingredients

Allergens

RECIPE:

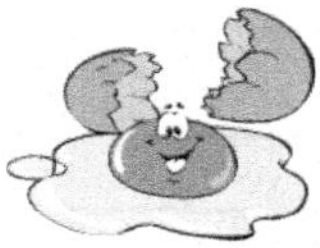

Cooking Instructions

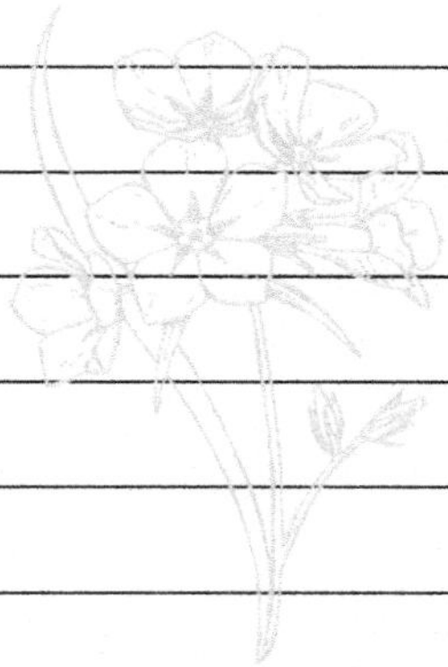

Ingredients

Allergens

RECIPE:

Cooking Instructions

Ingredients

Allergens

RECIPE:

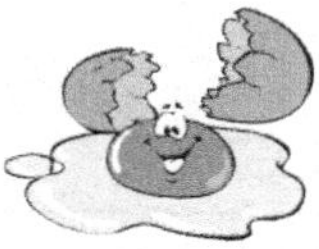

Cooking Instructions

Ingredients

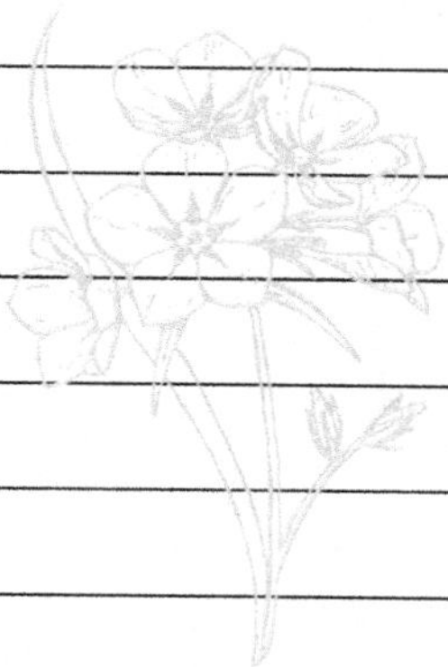

Allergens

RECIPE:

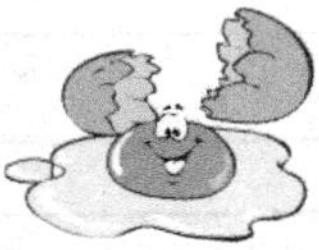

Cooking Instructions

Ingredients

Allergens

RECIPE:

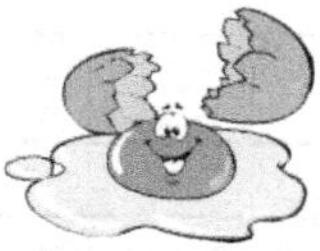

Cooking Instructions

Ingredients

Allergens

RECIPE:

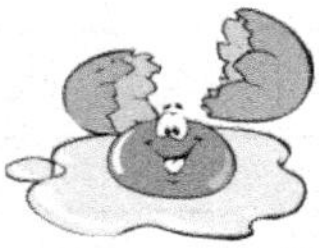

Cooking Instructions

Ingredients

Allergens

RECIPE:

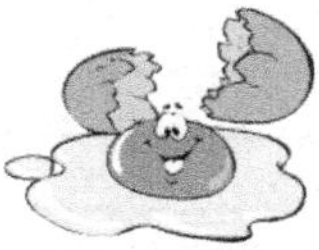

Cooking Instructions

Ingredients

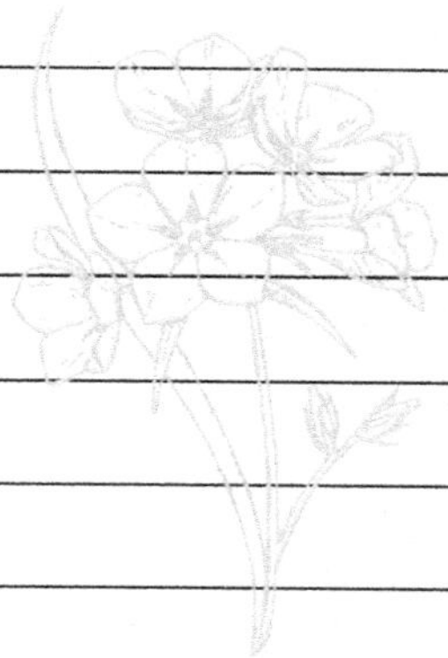

Allergens

RECIPE:

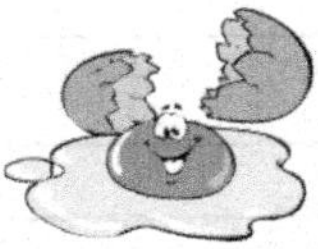

Cooking Instructions

Ingredients

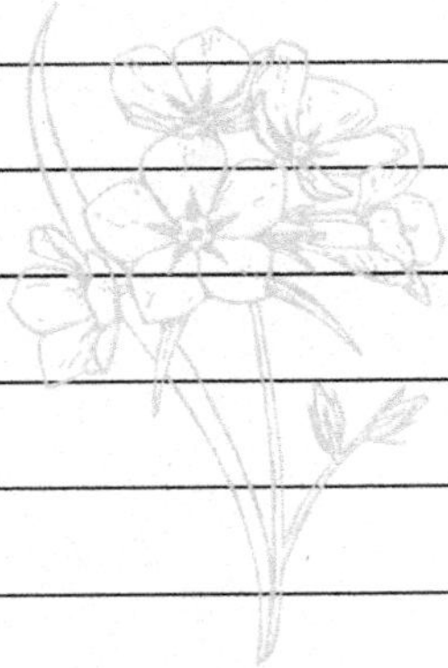

Allergens

RECIPE:

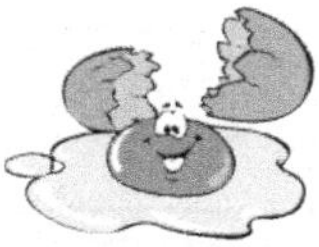

Cooking Instructions

Ingredients

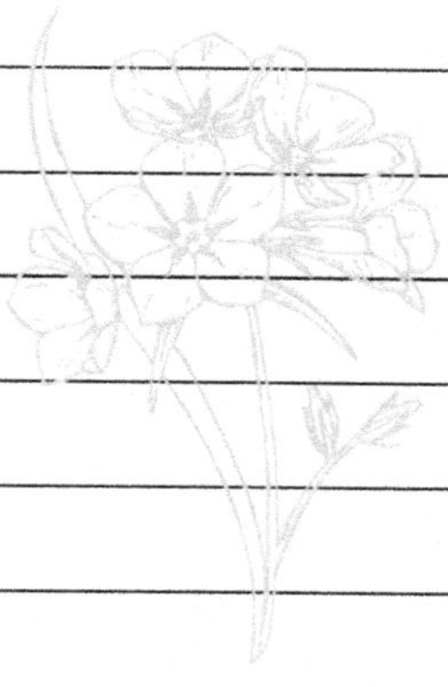

Allergens

RECIPE:

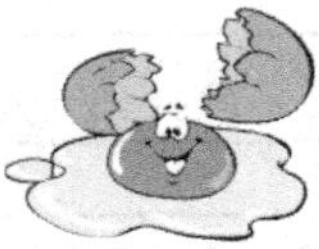

Cooking Instructions

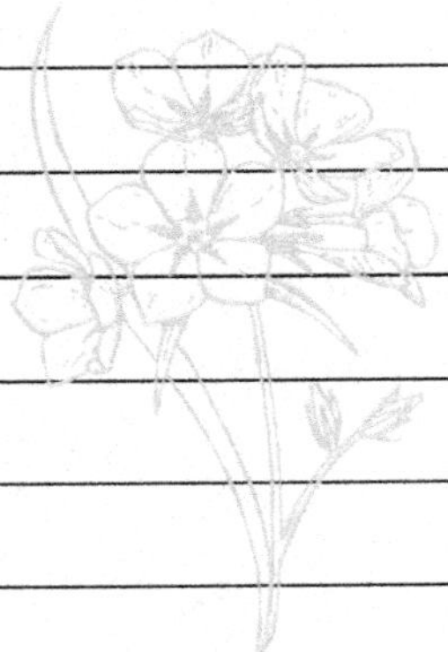

Ingredients

Allergens

RECIPE:

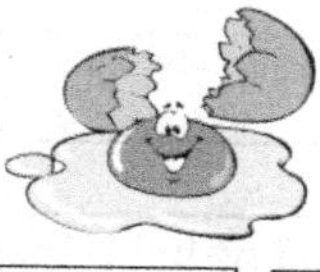

Cooking Instructions

Ingredients

Allergens

RECIPE:

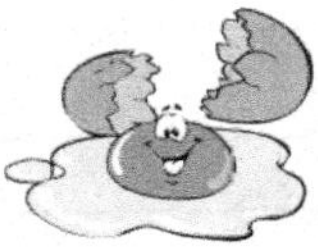

Cooking Instructions

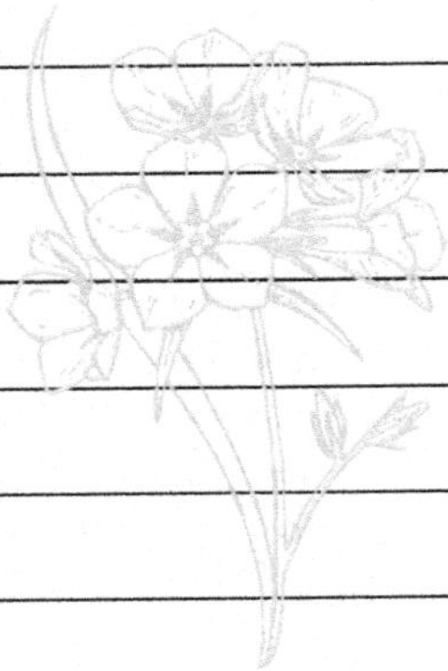

Ingredients

Allergens

RECIPE:

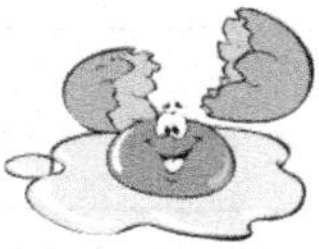

Cooking Instructions

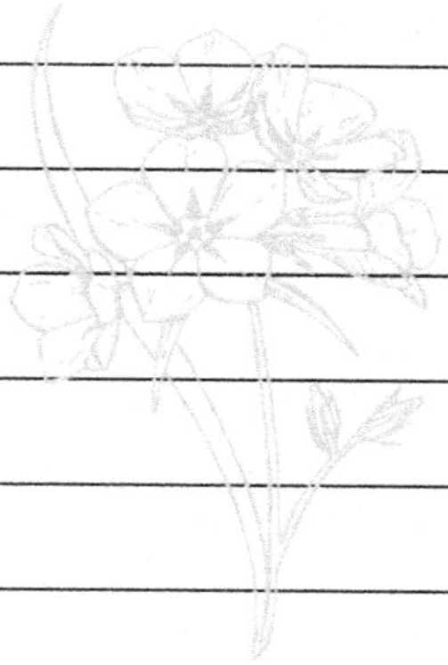

Ingredients

Allergens

RECIPE:

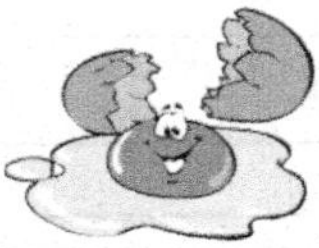

Cooking Instructions

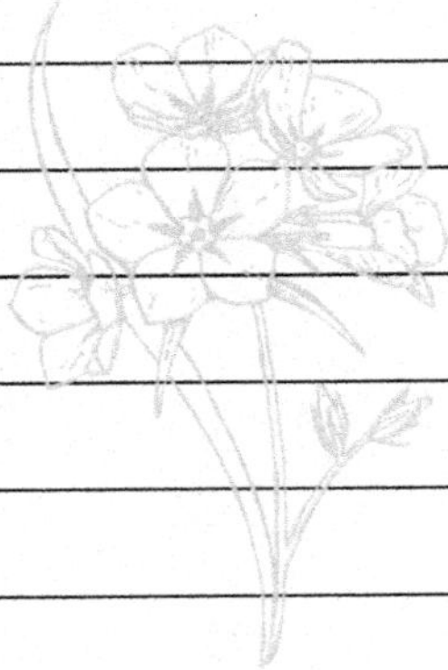

Ingredients

Allergens

RECIPE:

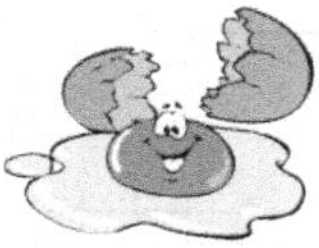

Cooking Instructions

Ingredients

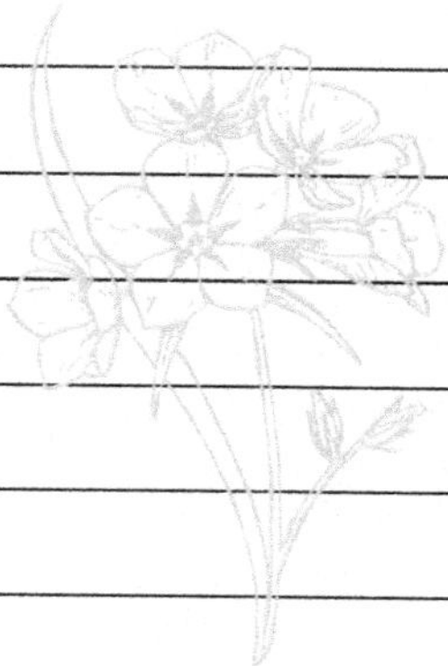

Allergens

RECIPE:

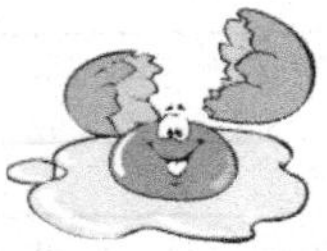

Cooking Instructions

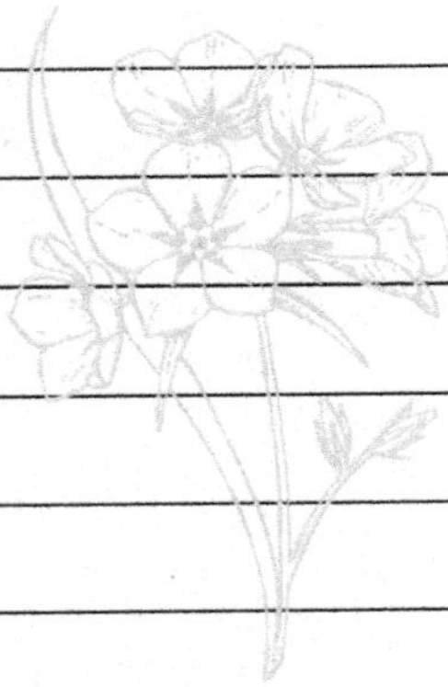

Ingredients

Allergens

RECIPE:

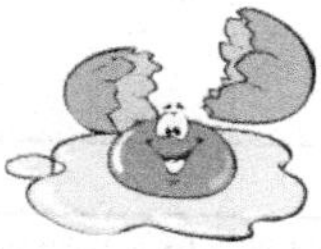

Cooking Instructions

Ingredients

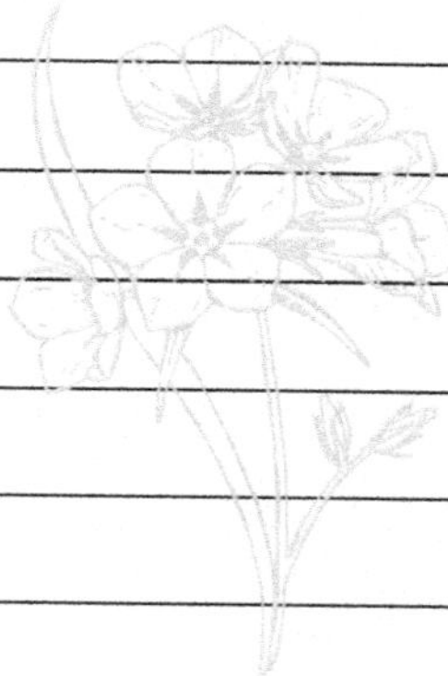

Allergens

RECIPE:

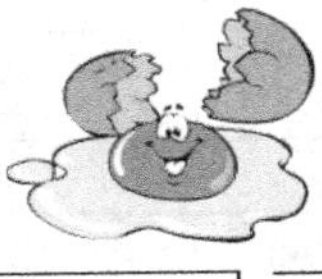

Cooking Instructions

Ingredients

Allergens

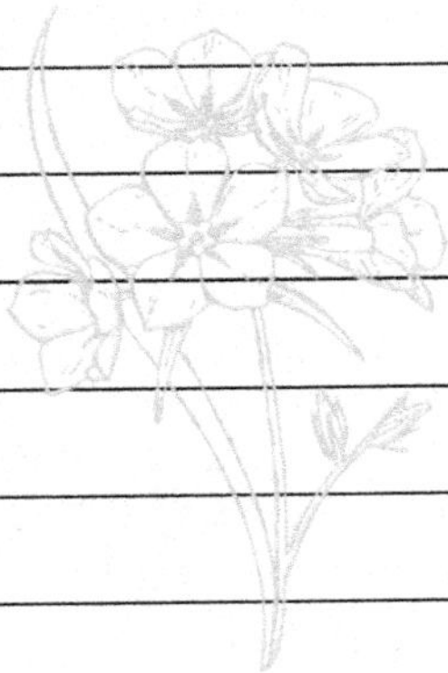

RECIPE:

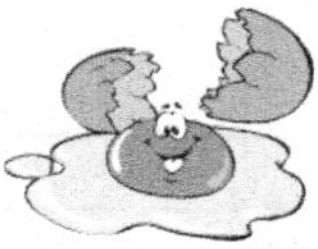

Cooking Instructions

Ingredients

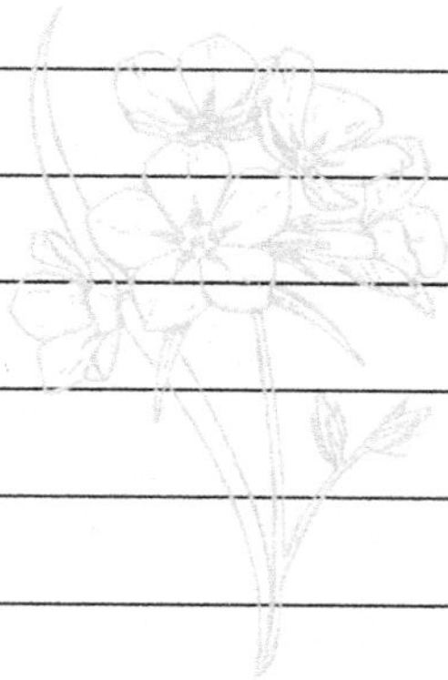

Allergens

RECIPE:

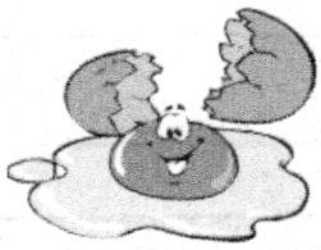

Cooking Instructions

Ingredients

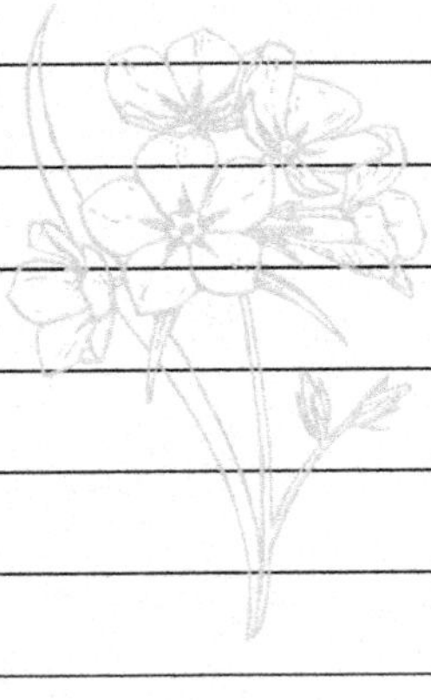

Allergens

RECIPE:

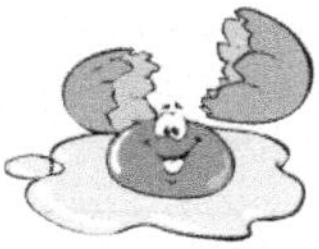

Cooking Instructions

Ingredients

Allergens

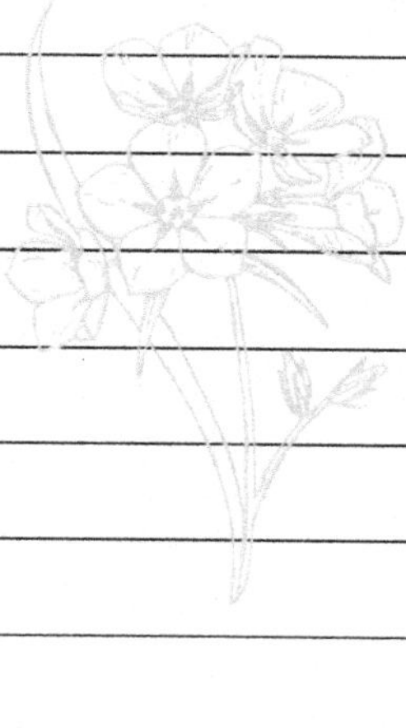

RECIPE:

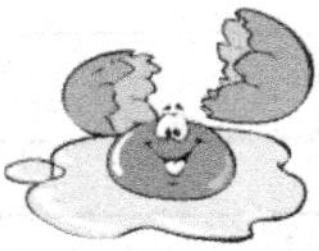

Cooking Instructions

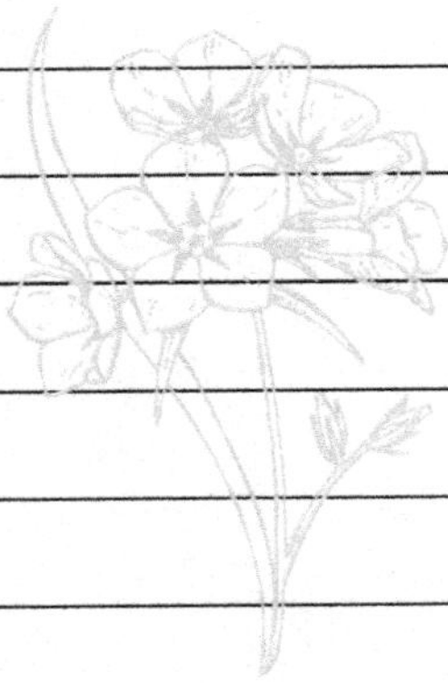

Ingredients

Allergens

RECIPE:

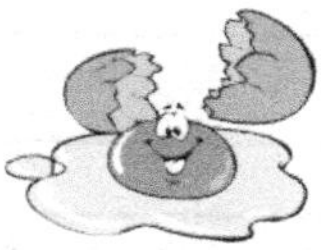

Cooking Instructions

Ingredients

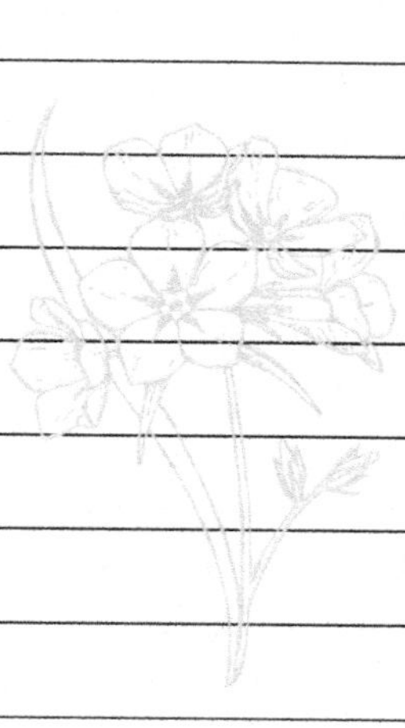

Allergens

RECIPE:

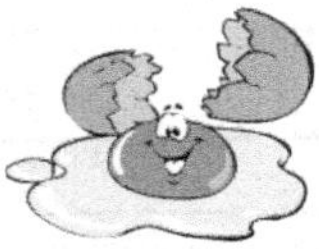

Cooking Instructions

Ingredients

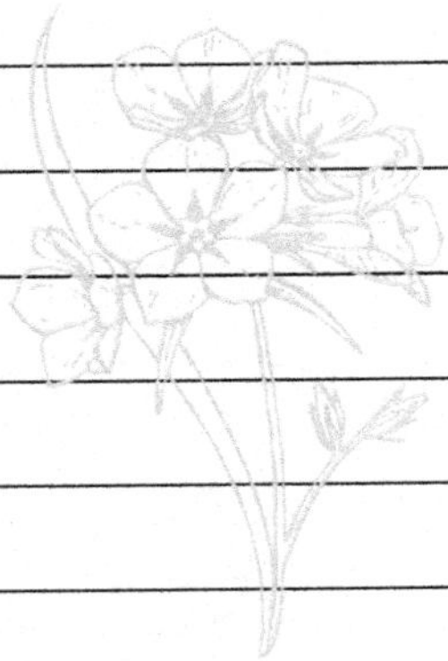

Allergens

RECIPE:

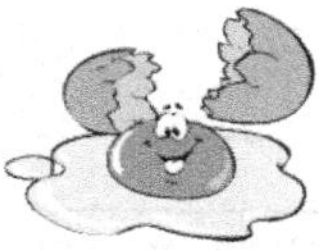

Cooking Instructions

Ingredients

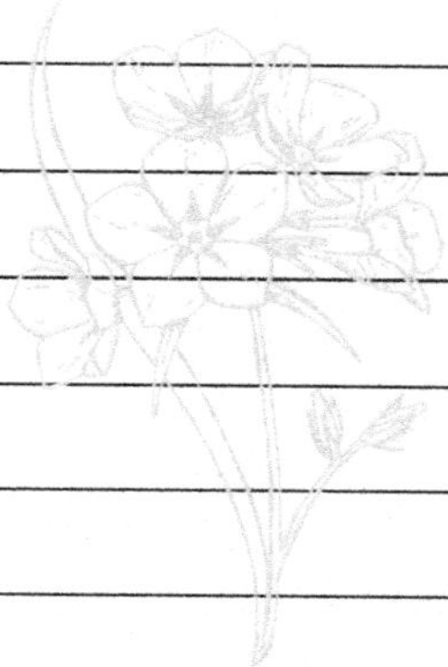

Allergens

RECIPE:

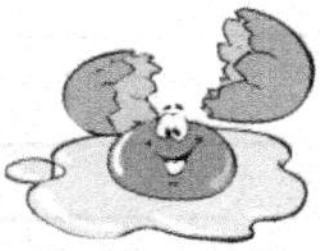

Cooking Instructions

Ingredients

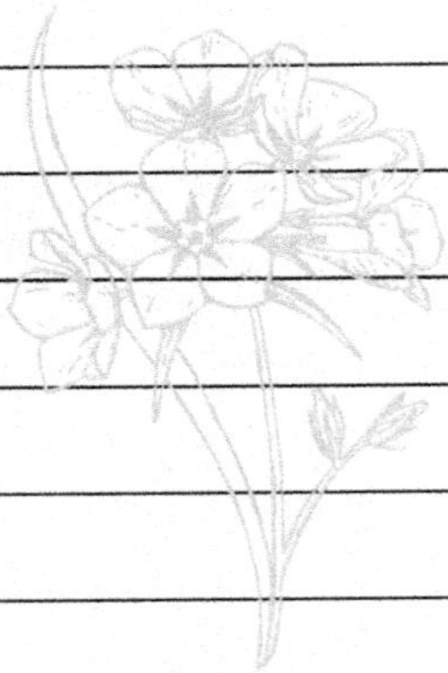

Allergens

RECIPE:

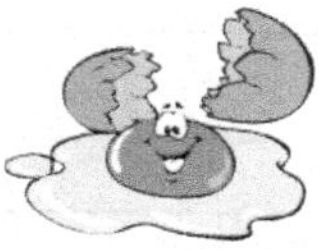

Cooking Instructions

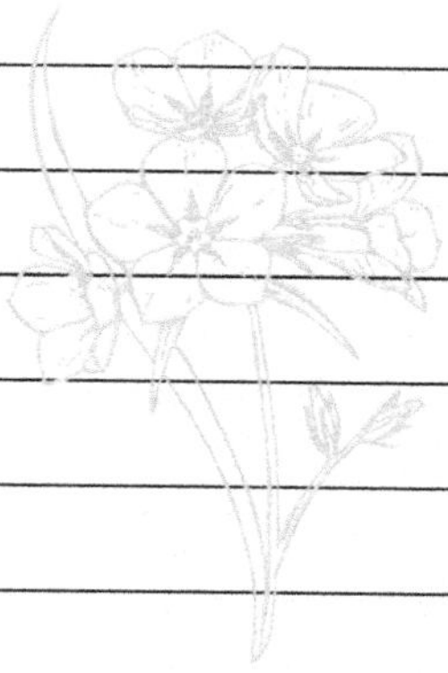

Ingredients

Allergens

RECIPE:

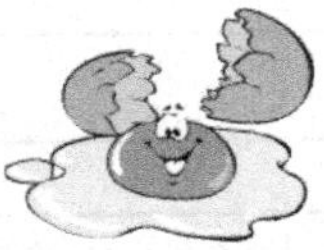

Cooking Instructions

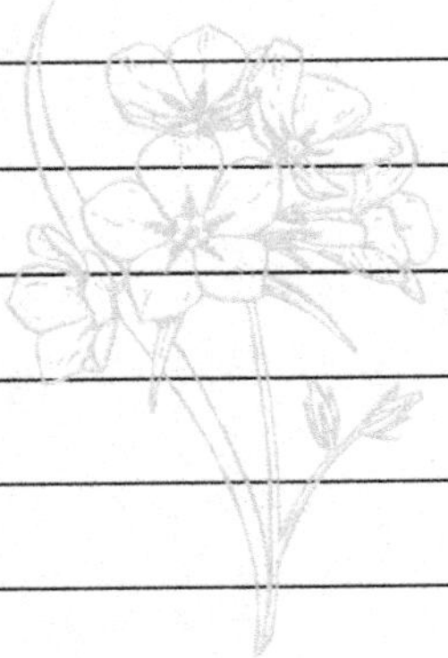

Ingredients

Allergens

RECIPE:

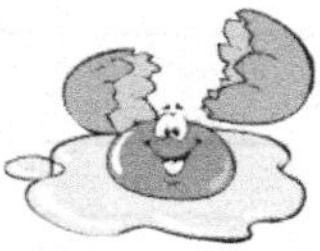

Cooking Instructions

Ingredients

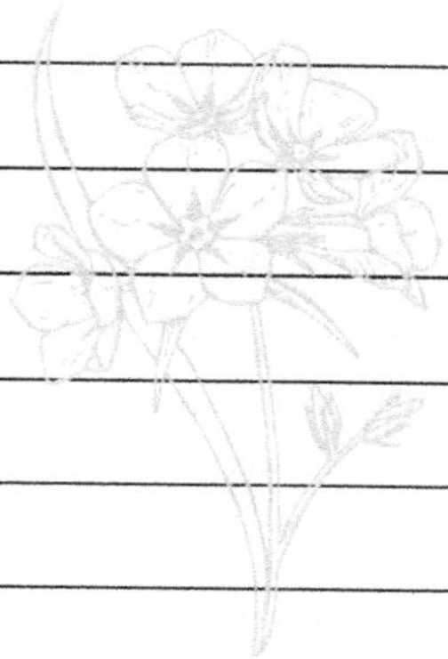

Allergens

RECIPE:

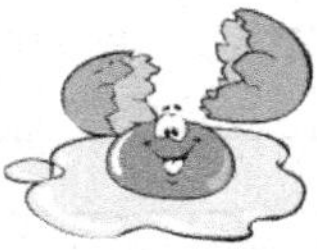

Cooking Instructions

Ingredients

Allergens

RECIPE:

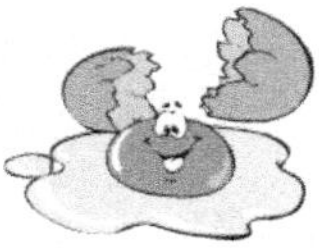

Cooking Instructions

Ingredients

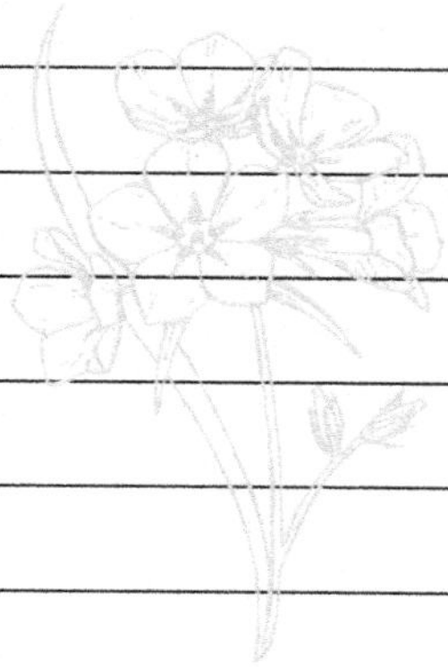

Allergens

Made in the USA
Monee, IL
04 November 2026

67383831R00059